Live, Laugh, LEAVE ME ALONE

HARPER FORD

avon.

Published by AVON
A division of HarperCollins*Publishers* Ltd
1 London Bridge Street
London SE1 9GF

www.harpercollins.co.uk

HarperCollins*Publishers*
Macken House, 39/40 Mayor Street Upper
Dublin 1, D01 C9W8, Ireland

A Paperback Original 2025
1

A catalogue record for this book is available from the British Library.

ISBN: 9780008763091

This novel is entirely a work of fiction. The names, characters and incidents portrayed in it are the work of the author's imagination. Any resemblance to actual persons, living or dead, events or localities is entirely coincidental.

Set in Sabon LT Std by HarperCollins*Publishers* India

Printed and bound in the UK using 100% Renewable
Electricity at CPI Group (UK) Ltd

This book contains FSC™ certified paper and other controlled sources to ensure responsible forest management.

For more information visit: www.harpercollins.co.uk/green

This story is dedicated to Janey Stevens, for her kindness and luminosity, for supporting my books since the beginning and always approaching the world with love and light.

Chapter 1

We wanted to be adults so bloody badly when we were kids, didn't we? Well, fuck a duck, look at us now. Miserable! We're all sodding miserable. Born in the seventies, endured puberty in the eighties, partied in the nineties – I don't know about you but I spent most of my childhood gazing longingly at the adult world and wanting to be a part of it so much, it made my gut ache. I remember sitting in the back of my mum's car while she drove us home through town at night, seeing random windows lit up mysteriously in houses or tower blocks, imagining the lives of the people who lived behind those yellow rectangles, people I'd never know or meet. They were exotic because they were grown-ups, living in their own houses, living fascinating lives. I couldn't bloody *wait* to be like them. But nobody tells you, do they, how the vast majority of adulthood is just . . . hassle. Constant hassle. And responsibility. And full of . . . people. Urgh. I mean, I used to like people, when I was a kid. I was quite gregarious, by all accounts. I wanted friends, family and fellas in my life. It kind of seemed like the whole point of life, really. Socialising, that is. Then work happened. Jobs and tasks and wages and tax and all that jazz. And I thought it meant freedom. It did, in a way. I escaped from home and never went back.

But then, I bet you've found this in your own work life – you're in this office and with these people you didn't choose to be with and what's more, you realise you're going to spend far more time with these people than your own spouse and kids, if you have them, and certainly far more than with your friends, who you see less and less and less as there's always a gazillion things you have to do and organise and you find yourself messaging friends or in group chats saying, *Yeah, let's get together! I'll be free in about . . . seventeen months' time?* So, you're forced to make a work family, because you certainly see them more than your own. But there's a big difference between work families and home families and that's hierarchy. Yeah, maybe your older sibling, if you have one, lords it over you as the eldest child, even when you're in your forties or whatever. And maybe your parents still scold you about not getting your car tyres checked often enough or that jumper you keep wearing that makes you look fat. But you can tell them to shove it. You could even tell them to fuck off, if you really wanted to. But not at work . . . and especially not if you're in charge of HR, like me.

I'm Lucy but you can call me Lu, like my friends do. Or rather, like my friend – singular – does. I've only really got one friend, my bestie, Jacqui. She's a journalist at the local newspaper and I've known her since school. We just always clicked. And she lives near me in Tunbridge Wells too. So we stuck together, come rain or shine. Other than that, I have colleagues. And they generally call me Lucy. So do my family, except my nephews, who found Lu easier from their infant days and it just stuck. My family, who I never see . . . (but more on them later). I've just realised I've started this story with a massive rant. Sorry about that. Actually, I'm not sorry about that. Something tells me you understand, you identify and maybe you even fancy having a massive rant as well. But before we go on with the ranting, let me set the scene for you a bit, so I'm not just this moany old cow with no context.

So, I'm Lu, I'm fifty-three years of age and I'm the director of HR at a family-owned insurance company in Tonbridge, Kent. I've worked my way up from an entry-level job at this company thirty long years ago. I live in a village on the outskirts of Tunbridge Wells called Rusthall, near a big lump of stone called Toad Rock because it's a rock and it looks like a toad. Strange claim to fame, I know, but there you are. I live in a nice, terraced house a couple of minutes from Toad Rock (I know, it sounds like a mixture between *Wind in the Willows* and *The Muppets*, but it's not nearly so picturesque, or fun). I was married once to a nice enough man, Martin. Married for nineteen years, together for twenty-four years. Then about six years ago, we realised we were bored. Just absolutely, mind-numbingly bored of each other. He was a good chap, no animosity, no arguments over the record collection (yes, we still had a load of vinyl and I let him take it all, probably stupidly, as it may well be worth a hell of a lot of money these days). And we sold our rather sizeable house in Borough Green, a nice little town near Sevenoaks, and I moved back to Tunbridge Wells, where I grew up. I don't know why I did that really. I don't know anyone here except Jacqui, not anymore. No family here either (again, more on that later). Maybe I moved back to Tunbridge Wells because it was familiar, because it had the patina of home. Maybe I was scared. I think I probably was, though I'd hate to admit it to myself. I've always been a fighter, me. Determined and driven, that was what my school reports said, at least the ones that saw my potential. The teachers who didn't like me called me stubborn and pig-headed. Well, screw them. I'm a director on a very decent wage with quite a bit stashed away in savings for a rainy day. What I'm going to do with those savings on a rainy day, I don't have a clue, but they're there nonetheless. So, that's me.

As I say, I've been at this company – Beane & Co Family Insurance – for most of my adult life. I started as an admin assistant not long after finishing a history degree at Canterbury, which proved to be probably the most useless uni subject after English in terms of getting a job anywhere. I applied for over fifty jobs that summer after I finished my exams. And only got one interview, at Beane & Co. And they took me on, bless them. I did filing for a while, answering phones and making coffee, that kind of thing. Then a little step up to senior admin assistant. I knuckled down and worked my way diligently up the company ladder. I wanted to make a success of myself and I was forever grateful to Beane & Co for giving me that chance. And the rest is . . . well, history, I suppose – though I never used a single thing I learnt in that degree in my professional life, apart from understanding how Thomas Cromwell felt working for King Henry VIII, serving a capricious master and making himself the enemy of all he dealt with. That's what it's like being in charge of HR; in short, everybody hates me. Or if they don't hate me, they fear me. Which turns to hate, sooner or later. Better fear than love, as Machiavelli advised. And even if they don't hate me, they can't be themselves around me, because I'm a spy for the directors, in their minds anyway. So I don't get invited to drinks or dinners or even lunch. And even if I did, I probably wouldn't go anyway, because the moment I walk in the pub, everyone shuts up as they'll have been slagging off their bosses and once I'm there, they can't do that anymore. Nobody confides in me, as a mate, I mean. So, as I moved up the company ladder, and into HR, and to the top of HR, and up to the directors' level, work friendships fell by the wayside and were never found again. So, here I am, top of the heap and I'm . . . well, the truth is, I'm lonely. Really lonely. Lonely as a little petunia in an onion patch, as the old song goes. But I suspect I'm more like an onion in a petunia patch.

Look, don't start feeling sorry for me. I can't stand pity. Can you? I mean, it's just shitty, isn't it, pity? When someone's looking at you that way, all sympathetic about poor old you, knowing full well in their head that they're not in your position, that they have a much nicer existence than you and although they're being nice, they're certainly glad they're not you. Well, for a start, I have a perfectly nice existence, all right? I'm bloody good at my job, I see my bestie regularly and I like where I live. Royal Tunbridge Wells is gorgeous. We have the Pantiles, the stunning little area of cobbled paths leading to charming shops and cafés, with festivals of antiques or gin and jazz. Plus, a little drive takes you to Scotney Castle and Bewl Water and other pretty places. I like TV documentaries about history and podcasts about history and I read history books. I like walking around stately homes and National Trust gardens and I go and do that kind of thing regularly. And I go on holiday alone, but that's what I prefer, because then you don't have to put up with other people's bollocks all the time (figuratively, not literally. I haven't had anything to do with a pair of bollocks in six years or more. And that suits me just fine, thanks). You're probably wondering, why hasn't she got a bloke? Because that's what people wonder about people like me. I did have a bloke, my ex-husband Martin. I had a nice one for nearly a quarter of a century. And no kids to complicate matters, as we both knew it wasn't for us. We met in my final year at Canterbury and he was doing Archaeology and we bonded over ancient ruins . . . that was, until our love life became ancient ruins. We were more like sister and brother by the end, me and Martin. And he wanted more than that and I didn't want to give it to him. Never been interested in all that stuff, really. And it just became sad somehow. Too sad to keep doing it. I never had a brother and I liked having a surrogate one for such a long time. I had a sister, I still do. But she was always bossy, though she's younger than me. She was forever my mum's favourite and I was my dad's, until we lost him. Not literally, we didn't misplace him like your birth certificate or a blouse you haven't seen in the wash for a while. It's a rather pointless euphemism for the fact that my dad died. And I lost my best mate, my defender, my cheerleader, my champion. (Anyway, more on that later.)

So, at work, the director of HR has this weird in-between existence, where you're serving the CEO and the other directors, while you're also representing the rank and file, fighting their battles for them. But also you're disciplining them. So you're good cop and bad cop all in one. And that's why nobody trusts you, because you serve two masters: the staff and the management. Honestly, heading up HR is probably the loneliest job on the planet; even lighthouse keepers can see their mates whenever they're on leave and everybody trusts them, because they save ships and other heroic and picturesque things. The director of HR has no such glamour. And no support either. I'm looking after everyone else's interests at work. But who's looking after mine? Nobody, that's who. I've known this for years but I've never felt so crappy about it until recently. I just don't want this job anymore. Truth be told, I don't want anything more to do with HR ever. Don't get me wrong: I want to stay in this company. I've worked my way up from nothing to a high level here and I'm not willing to throw all that away and start all over again somewhere new. God no. Too old for that. I just don't want to deal with people. They're just so bloody . . . peopley. What I really want – what I'd love – is if this company created the post of COO, that is, chief operating officer. I want to focus on operations, not people. I have the knowledge and expertise for it, I just know I do. Beane & Co doesn't have a COO, as such. Never has. Those responsibilities have been managed for decades by various directors between them. But there have been rumblings in recent years that the CEO will create a COO role soon, though nothing has transpired. I've had my hopes up for far too long. I've spent all my adult years working for this company – it's been my life in many ways. I'm grateful to it, I'm loyal to it and I've worked my way up and want to finish my career here too, at the top of the heap. I could leave, I could seek out a COO post elsewhere but there's something in me that feels that would be failure. I've worked my backside off to attain the highest level at this company I've given so much of my life to and there's no way I'm leaving while there's still a chance of the post I've always wanted. So here I am, still waiting. And in the meantime, I have to deal with this lot: people. Staff. The minions below snapping at my heels, the managers above pouring their buckets of slop on my head. It's an uncomfortable position, as I'm sure you can appreciate, about as easy as sleeping on Lego.

It really came home to me how much I'm beginning to detest being the face of HR these days, when I was running a dreaded staff training session. Oh God, I hate staff training with a loathing that is brighter than the fucking sun. Everybody hates it, don't they? Does anyone wake up on a staff training day and leap out of bed in glorious anticipation? No, they bloody don't. They moan and groan their way into the training room and look at me when they enter the room like I ran over their cat in my 4X4 and then reversed back over it just for shits and giggles. So, there I am, last Tuesday – it must be the most horrible day of the week, mustn't it, Tuesday? Monday, you're just in survival mode. Wednesday is hump day, so you're heading nearer to the end of the week than you were. Tuesday is that shitty little day in the middle of the beginning of the week, that seems like you're still in the foothills of Everest and yet you're feeling like crap already and still have eight thousand metres to go. And this particularly awful Tuesday where I had to deliver training to the troops was on a particularly deadly subject and that was 'general behaviours'. Yes, that's what we have to call it. And though its title may be bland, buckle up, because you're about to enter the ridiculous, rage-inducing world of HR bullshit doublespeak.

'So, general behaviours,' I begin, to the thirty or so reluctant spectators in the training room (and yes, that's not the whole company, so I will have to do the whole thing again several times before I'm done with 'general behaviours').

'These include all of those indeterminate actions that go on at work that aren't included in other policies but could become problematic.'

Everybody's looking at me like I've interrupted their favourite show with an advert about laxatives.

'What we're focusing on here is behaviours around the office that, although seemingly harmless, may well be causing offence to others.'

At this point, several people audibly sigh. And I'm sure I hear loudmouth Lorraine from Accounts say the word 'woke'. But I must soldier on.

'This could be, for example, using inappropriate language around the office. Engaging in inappropriate banter. Bringing in personal items, such as mugs or notebooks, or even wearing certain items of clothing, with inappropriate language on. To continue the clothing theme, let's remember that we've introduced our more casual dress code recently, due to staff demand. And this has worked well for the most part, yet certain items of clothing have, I'm afraid, gone too far, such as crop tops, activewear and yes, even pyjamas, or at least trousers that look suspiciously like pyjamas. And even some of those who've dressed more smartly for work have chosen to come to the office with wording on their T-shirts that has caused offence to others.'

'Like what?' calls out Lorraine.

I knew she'd pipe up. She always does. She's got an opinion on every damn thing on God's green earth. The toilets, the snack bar, the water beakers, the lifts, the antibacterial spray in the coffee area, for fuck's sake. Every. Damn. Thing.

'Sorry, Lorraine?' I say, smiling politely. 'What kind of example did you want?'

'What wording on T-shirts is offensive? I haven't seen anyone with an offensive T-shirt. Give us one example of one T-shirt that somebody in this office has worn to work that you think is offensive. Go on!'

A ripple of expectation goes around the group, all waiting for me to prove my point.

Jesus Christ, I want to pick up this dreary and unimaginative office chair I'm seated on and hurl it at her stupid, belligerent face.

'I'm sure you can understand, Lorraine, that it's not about what I personally find offensive.'

I want to say, *For example, I would not find it offensive if the caretaker came in and punched your teeth down your throat, Lorraine.* But obviously, I can't say that.

'It's a judgement call about what's appropriate for a professional environment. I can't give you exact examples, as that would single out specific members of staff and I'm not going to do that. But I will say that anything that involves the word "pussy" and is not about cats is probably a bad idea. The same goes for "cock" and game birds, "bitch" and female canines and even, on one memorable occasion, a four-letter word that the venerated Chaucer used in his famous work *The Canterbury Tales* and yet is most likely an ill-advised choice for a staff meeting, the first letter being *C* and the remainder of the words comprising the one-syllable *UNT*.'

A titter emanates from the mob. And they are looking more to me like a mob, a sinister gathering of individuals who've got it in for me. There are one or two shy people at the sides who don't hate me and are sitting up, keenly listening and nodding. Bless their cotton socks. But the rest of them are brooding, and shaking their heads, or rolling their eyes, or squaring up for outright attack, like bloody Lorraine from Accounts.

Lorraine says, 'And why is it offensive? Nobody's saying it out loud. Nobody's going over to Glenda from Finance and calling her a C U Next Tuesday, are they? Why can't you lot take a joke?'

'Yeah!' cries bolshy Barry from Sales, with gusto. 'If it's written down, how's it going to hurt someone? Sticks and stones, and all that! How the hell are written-down words going to cause trouble or hurt someone?'

'*Mein Kampf* springs to mind,' I say under my breath, and immediately regret it as most who heard it are looking confused but the ones who get the reference are a bit shocked. And unfortunately, though Barry from Sales usually would not be able to locate his way out of a paper bag, he must be into war films or something, because he does indeed get the reference.

'You calling me a Nazi?!' splutters Barry.

'If anyone's a Nazi round here . . . ' adds Lorraine, trailing off and folding her arms triumphantly, nodding in my direction, which solicits a general muttering of agreement.

'Oh, fuck the lot of you! Do you think I give a flying fart what puerile slogan you tedious wankers wear on your armpit-stained bought-off-a-Facebook-ad bleached-out-cheap-as-chips-shitty-fabric T-shirt to work? DO YOU?'

Of course, I don't say this. I'm a professional. Instead, I have to persevere in this ridiculous charade for the next twenty-seven minutes, feeling more and more like the wildebeest on a David Attenborough documentary surrounded by ravenous hyenas. I'm standing there, in the middle of all this invective, thinking to myself, when did people become so utterly shit?

Have they always been shit and I just had more optimism, or more patience? Because right now, I'm telling you, given the choice of listening to these bastards hurl abuse at me just for the presumption of doing my damn job, I'd rather douse the office in petrol and burn the whole fucking thing to the ground.

Chapter 2

My name is Lucy Cooper and I'm a workaholic. Yes, I may as well get it out there. But the thing is, whereas alcoholics get a bad name, I see my condition as a strength. And also it's a choice, not a compulsion. My ex-husband told me I was a workaholic as if it were a bad thing. All right, I probably eat too much junk food and drink too much wine, but other than that, I'd say my work-life balance is just right: ninety per cent work, ten per cent life. Work fills my life, mostly, and I'm very happy about that, thank you very much. I'm bloody good at my job, because I work my arse off to make it good. If only I could get rid of these pesky people I have to manage, I'd actually be happy in my job too, as well as being good at it. I used to have far more patience for people than I do now, that is true. These days, people rub me up the wrong way. Must be something to do with hitting your fifties. Your stock of patience has been dwindling for a while then – BOOM – one day, you realise it's bottomed out. Zero patience remaining. Look, I know being COO doesn't mean I won't have anything to do with human beings. Part of my role will be to manage the needs of my workforce, but I won't be so hands on. I'll be largely managing strategy, expansion and other juicy things like that. I'm ready for it. Nothing stands in my way.

So, you can imagine my delight at what happens next. Not in that training session with loudmouth Lorraine and bolshy Barry, which descended further into the seventh circle of hell once we started talking about why nobody should be mentioning nipples in a sales meeting. No, this happens a few days later, this morning in fact, at our weekly directors' meeting. Firstly, let me introduce you to our CEO. He's called Derek, he's fifteen years older than me and he's best friends with our lord and master Gerald Beane, who owns the company inherited from his now deceased father Gerard Beane. (That's not a typo. The dad was Gerard, with an R, and the son Gerald, with an L. I mean, why call your kid nearly the same name as you bar one letter? That's just asking for trouble when it comes to opening letters on the hall table.) Mr Beane (I know . . .) lives in a villa in Spain and is about as interested in the day-to-day running of his company as a fish is a bicycle. Derek's been doing this job for the last twenty-three years and everyone's been expecting him to retire for about a decade, since he started leaving earlier and earlier on Fridays for golf until eventually he left the office on a Thursday after lunch and hasn't done a Friday in donkey's years. I get on all right with Derek, I suppose. He's not a bad person, just slightly . . . what's the term . . . old school? Okay, that's far too generous. Chauvinistic? Truth is, he's sexist and cloth-eared about any social movements beyond around 1950. But he understands money and he knows the insurance business inside out. He looks like a mixture between Bob

Hope (the nose) and Leslie Nielsen (the towering side-parting of gleaming white hair and year-round tan). And today, Derek has an announcement to make.

'All right, troops, at ease,' he begins. The seven directors – six men and one woman, i.e. me – are seated around the oval table in the conference room, and Derek is standing before a large, framed photograph of himself with Gerald Beane on the wall, dressed in grey suits at some dreary awards ceremony about twenty years ago, both with brown hair and about three stone lighter. 'Time for an announcement. I know I haven't laid the groundwork for this and it'll come like a bolt from the blue but I'm retiring. There it is. I'll be staying another three months or so until the annual staff conference at the end of March, which will be my last official day of engagement. After that, I'm off to pastures new! Namely, to the place where the rain falls mainly on the plain.'

Some of the younger directors won't get this reference, but I used to spend Sunday afternoons on the sofa with my dad watching old movies and I know all about the rain falling mainly on the plain in Spain, as our favourites were old musicals like *My Fair Lady*. So . . . Derek is off to Spain. His wife Janey has wanted to go for ages. Poor Janey. She's a lovely woman, is Janey. And far too good for him. I've met her at staff dos before and she always comes across as tolerant of him but a bit jaded. I've heard she's been hassling him to move out to Spain for the past few years to their swanky villa down the road from Mr and Mrs Beane in their swanky villa, so it was about time our CEO hit the road. I cannot describe to you the joy I feel at hearing this news. Because once Derek's gone, then we'll be getting a newer, and hopefully younger, CEO. One who's more with it, one who doesn't ignore half of my suggestions because I'm the only female amongst the directors, one I can talk into creating a COO post. And giving said post to me.

An undulation of congratulations goes around the table, some directors standing up to shake Derek's hand. A couple have started an impromptu round of applause, which dies down pretty smartish. I'm sitting there with a grin on my face. This is it. Now is my time! I can't wait to hear more. I can't wait to meet the new guy. (And it will be a guy. It's always a guy. You know how long I've been here. And I'm the first and only woman at this level in all that time.) I'm eager for Derek to tell us more.

'I'm hoping for a smooth transition, folks. And that's why Gerry B and myself have come up with a solution that will make it as straightforward as possible, and that's that the new CEO will be in and out of the office over the next few weeks or so to lubricate the gears and ease you all friction-free into the new regime. My worthy successor, a brand-new CEO, has already been appointed by Gerry and is quite the impressive chap, even though he is apparently coming from that unfamiliar territory beyond the Watford Gap, namely, the north. I believe he hails originally from Grimsby, that godforsaken place by all accounts, but don't hold that against him. He has also lived and worked in the United States, so I'm sure he'll be full of bright and shiny new ideas from the new world. He's going to be popping in this afternoon, along with . . . well, let's leave that little nugget of information aside for the moment. More about that anon. Firstly, I'd like to thank you all for . . . '

And off he goes on a lengthy account of his thousands of days spent at Beane & Co, which I won't relay to you because, honestly, you'd throw this book in the hotel pool, or out of the train window, or send it sailing into the bin wherever you happen to be reading it. I have to sit through this tedious nonsense, but lucky you, you don't. After the meeting, once more handshakes and back-slapping have taken place, I manage to get a minute alone with Derek. I don't mess about.

'Will the new CEO be creating a COO post, Derek?'

Derek smiles and wags his finger at me, which makes me want to snap it off at the knuckle. But I resist.

'A little bird has told me that this may well be on the cards, Lucia.'

My name is not Lucia. You know that. And Derek knows that. But because I have dark eyes and used to have a pretty impressive mane of black hair before I hacked it all off. (These days I sport a swish grey bob, which I like, but nobody else seems to, especially my mother, who says I look like a 'chubby Helen Mirren' and I told her that was actually a huge compliment to which she replied, 'It wasn't meant to be', eyeing my middle-aged spread.) Derek has always presumed I'm Italian, despite me telling him that I'm not on numerous occasions. And thus has always called me Lucia, pronounced LOO-chia, with the totally incorrect-sounding stress on the first syllable, which also makes me want to punch him.

'That's good news,' I say. 'Any more information that you're willing to part with at this stage?'

'Now, now. Patience is a virtue. Wait until this afternoon. All will be revealed.'

He loves that, keeping us guessing. He's a keen game-player, is Derek, and not just of the golfing variety. So, the new CEO is in later plus someone else, is it? Derek was being his usual obtuse and infuriating self. I get through the rest of the morning with a lighter step, despite chairing a disciplinary over the manager of risk threatening her subordinate with a just-boiled kettle. Don't ask.

We reconvene at 2pm to meet the new guy (and it is of course a guy, as it always is and always has been amongst the directors of Beane & Co). The seven of us hover in anticipation in the conference room. I can tell some of the men in here are put out. They've developed their standing in the company nicely over the years and most of them were pretty convinced they had Derek wrapped around their little fingers. One or two of them may even have thought they'd be in with a chance of being named the new CEO. But one of the few bonuses of being in charge of HR is that the CEO regularly confides in me about who's winding him up and every single one of these blokes has rubbed him up the wrong way at one time or another. So, there's a heavy atmosphere of threatened testosterone in the room. What if this new CEO isn't as easy to manipulate as Derek? That's what I'm pretty sure they're thinking, as they shift about and keep glancing at the door. I'm just banking on getting a meeting with him ASAP, so I can float the COO idea immediately. I don't want anyone else suggesting it and throwing their hat in the ring before I can make my pitch.

Then, in comes Sharon, Derek's PA, and shows in the new guy. The first thing I think is – Gary Lineker. But not the silver fox of today, instead the one from about twenty years ago. Tall, greying hair yet still some dark bits, in a cropped style and a big smile with white teeth. A shiny young Gary Lineker, even though this guy comes from Grimsby. And he's young, I mean, younger than anyone in this room by a good few years. Early forties? I'd guess forty-three. I'm very good at nailing down ages. Been working with people too long. So, Gary Lineker steps aside and behind him, inexplicably, is a woman. It's so weird to see another woman coming into the directors' conference room other than Sharon, that I'm quite discombobulated. And this one is definitely not a Sharon, definitely not an assistant. She looks younger than me at first glance, much younger, but another few quick glances in her direction confirm she's not far off my age. I'd say . . . hmm . . . forty-nine, on the terrifying cusp of her fifties (though not terrifying for me. I couldn't wait to be fifty and have people's expectations about my appearance slide down the slippery slope to late female middle-age and general invisibility). She's about a foot taller than me in steely high heels (a direct contrast to my comfy yet classic Clarks shoes), with what I would call a power haircut. We've both got short bobs but there the similarity ends. Hers is a deep natural-looking red with straight lines across the fringe, back and sides that look like they were ruled with an electron microscope. She clocks me immediately and looks away, no smile. Okay . . . what's going on here?

We all sidle somewhat uncomfortably to our chairs as Derek seats Gary Lineker and Mary Quant either side of him. Derek is looking quite obsequious, a cringey new experience for him. He looks pleased with himself though, as if these two are his eldest offspring. He introduces them as Nick Bridges and Tara Harryman. He talks about their credentials, what companies they've worked for, what positions they've attained. They sit there with smiles plastered on their faces listening to this endless monologue. It must be hurting their facial muscles. Finally – *finally* – Derek finishes and it's Nick and Tara's turn to talk.

Look, I'm not going to bore you with their corporate-buzzword-infested speeches. Suffice to say, Nick is keen as mustard to 'renew and revamp' Beane & Co, which seemingly scares the hell out of the other directors if their terrified rictus smiles are anything to go by. I'm listening carefully because I'm looking for my way in with this shiny new CEO. I'm plotting, I'm planning, I'm awaiting my chance to nab him afterwards and raise the idea of a COO. It's certainly looking promising. I'm delighted this new bloke has turned up and is going to give this place a much needed kick up the backside. Then, it's time for Tara to speak and I'm agog. Who is this person? Nick introduces her.

'I'd like you all to welcome my right-hand person, my number one, my co-pilot!'

All right, get on with it, man. Enough politically correct denominations.

'Tara and I have worked together some years now, at CXGA and at BJ&Z . . .'

He says *zee*, like the Americans do. Is that really necessary? Is it, Nick?

'And now here at Beane & Co Tara joins us as director of legal services, a new role I've created for the company, as we both agreed that the management structure does need some tweaking. She'll be starting today and getting to grips with the business and reporting back to me, until I start my role proper in three months' time. So, please make her feel welcome and help her out with anything she needs to know. I'll be in and out of the office in the meantime, to smooth the transition. And let me assure you, I'm raring to go in this . . .'

You get the picture. It goes on like this for a while, with a list of new initiatives which piss us all off, as it'll mean more work for everyone. New people love creating new work for the old ones, don't they? It makes them look like they're doing something. Effecting change and all that LinkedIn bullshit. So, there we have it. The new guard. But Tara doesn't get a speech. She just sits there looking pleased with herself. She's enigmatic, she's got a scary hairdo, she's . . . well, I don't know for sure but – despite her scary hairdo – could this possibly be a female comrade, at long last, in the directors of Beane & Co? It would be rather fab to have another woman around here. I've been thinking that for years.

After all this formality, Sharon has clearly been instructed to bring in refreshments, as a few plates of M&S sandwiches and iced buns are ferried in, plus sparkling water. (Urgh. Does anyone actually like sparkling water? It tastes like wall.)

I ignore the food and head towards Nick. The other directors are all eager to talk to Tara. Yes, she looks good for her age but I reckon it's more about the other guys feeling less intimidated by her. Nick's white-toothed Gary Lineker glamour has put them all out. I don't care about any of that. I just want my promotion. I make a beeline for him and, after the requisite period of small talk, I go straight in for the kill.

'I've been suggesting changes in the management structure of Beane & Co for quite a while, Nick,' I manage to shoehorn in. 'The post of COO is conspicuous by its absence.'

There. It's out there.

'I totally agree with you there, Lucy. It's something I noticed straight away when analysing the company's structure. Tara spotted it too. We've been discussing it quite a bit. More on that soon. You're interested, I take it?'

'I am indeed.'

Job done. And I'm not going to blow it by oversharing my

real reason for wanting to be COO: that I fucking hate people and want to work with as few of them as possible. For now, I need him to know I'm ambitious and that's enough. We chat a bit more and then he calls over Tara. She immediately perks up at the sound of his voice and strides over quick smart. Nick introduces us. And then, we are face to face, the old guard of me in my Clarks shoes versus the new guard of Mary Quant. I mean, Tara. Even her name carries a hint of allure. I'd like to have a chat with her without this lot around, find out more about her, bond a bit with the second ever female director here. We could make quite the formidable team, given half a chance. I'm about to ask her a friendly yet professional question to get the ball rolling, when Derek appears and interrupts me, as usual.

'Ah, I can't tell you, Nick, and you two ladies as well, how pleasing it is for me to see another fine female in this conference room. I just know you two and Nick are going to shake this place up together. I'm guessing Lucia . . . '

STOP CALLING ME THAT! AAAAAAARRRGGGHHH!

'. . . has already mentioned the COO post to you, Nick? Yeah, I knew she would! She's been banging on about it for years! And now, you'll be thrilled to find out, Lucia, that Nick wants to appoint one the minute he starts. But don't get too excited, because you're not the only one who wants it, is she, Tara, eh? That's right, Lucia. Meet your lady rival, Tara! Hey, Nick, I'm looking forward to this particular mud fight, aren't you?'

Oh, FUCK.

Chapter 3

I'm on my sofa with a KitKat and glass of Montidori Sangiovese and I'm internet stalking Tara Harryman – even her name is interesting. Far more interesting than Lucy Cooper. I sound like a librarian and she sounds like an international spy. We didn't get much of a chance to speak today but tomorrow is her first full day at work and I've been asked by Derek to help her settle in. Something tells me she won't need my help.

I can't believe this is happening. After all these years, the job I've wanted more than anything is finally being dangled before my eyes and yet my view is completely dwarfed by an unforeseen rival of titanic proportions. It enrages me too that, as director of HR, I should've been intimately involved in the appointment of any new staff, yet this new CEO – Gary Lineker, I mean, Nick Bridges – brought her in without any discussion or approval. He can do what he likes, within reason, but still, it's really pissed me off. And thus the stage is set for the next few weeks: the showdown of the century, between me and Tara Harryman for my dream job. At work,

I'll have to pretend to be courteous and helpful. But inside, I'm sure that we both know we must become the best of frenemies. And I'm on it already, spying on Ms Harryman like a pro. Namely, I'm having a nose through her Facebook and LinkedIn profiles.

Urgh. Just urgh. The output on both platforms is exactly the same. I mean, precisely. Same photos, same text. Maybe she has a secret private Facebook page for friends and family, but this one is all business all of the time. It's not just stuff about work, yet every post seems crafted to make her seem like employee of the year. Endless aspirational photos of Tara like some kind of *#bossbabe*. She runs and does half-marathons – of course. She eats organic and has a vegan day once a week – of course. She has a stand-up desk at home with a treadmill underneath it – of course. Hashtags she uses include:

#selfcare – I'm sure you care more about yourself than anyone else, Tara.

#mindbodysoul – shut up.

#healthylifestyle – of course you have this (I say, wiping KitKat smears from my dressing gown lapel).

#selflove – again, shut up.

#balance – I don't think my two large glasses of wine tonight would bode well for my balance right now.

#wellness – there it is. That word. It's such a buzz word in corporate HR right now. Managing the wellness of our staff. Fuck, I loathe that word. It feels made up, doesn't it? Like, the opposite of illness is wellness. But it isn't, is it? The opposite of illness is . . . feeling normal. Feeling okay. Isn't that the best most of us can hope for? I don't know, but that wellness word has always rubbed me up the wrong way. It

stinks of moral virtue. I'm more well than you! Look at me! I'm so fucking well!

#wellnesswednesday – only once a week, Tara? Lazy.

#wellnesswarrior – oh FUCK RIGHT OFF.

There's a post from this afternoon about starting at Beane & Co, including a spontaneous selfie with Nick outside our office building, in front of the brass plaque old Gerry Beane put up there a few years back. It needs a good polish. Tara and Nick, however, look like what would happen if corporate androids took over the world. Hair, skin, outfit, smile – all absolutely on point. I look down at my dressing gown I'm wearing, over my work blouse and M&S knickers plus slipper socks. Does Tara ever dress like this at home? Does Tara ever relax from being so bloody perfect all the time? I sigh. I haven't thought to worry about my work appearance for years. Working with six directors, all male, meant that I learnt quickly to dress in a way that rendered my femininity undetectable. Nothing to mark me out as a woman. Nothing to mark me out as different from them. Slacks, plain blouses, flat shoes. Tara doesn't subscribe to this. I look down at her latest post on Facebook. It's from tonight. She's posted a picture of herself in activewear – of course – grinning at the camera with a big thumbs up. Stop grinning all the time, for fuck's sake. What's she talking about in this post, anyway? Has she run a cheeky little full marathon in between the office and home? Has she had a kale smoothie for her dinner? I glance at the remains of a Thai takeaway on the table that I got on the way home. It was so good. Not good *for* me, but good nonetheless. I bet Tara never gets takeaways, unless you count protein energy bars at her pricey gym. Then it hits me. Oh God, she's going to get this job. She's so bloody perfect and she's so far up the new CEO's arse, he's sure to pick her. I mean, she's just such an impressive person, in every way. Too perfect to bear. Whereas me . . . I have the years of experience and knowledge to smash this COO post. But we all know that when it comes to promotions, the world isn't quite the meritocracy we want it to be. Let's face it, I don't walk the walk and talk the talk and have the right hair, the right shoes or the right hashtags. Tara appears every part the killer career woman to power walk her way into Beane & Co's bright shiny future alongside silver fox Gary Lineker, whereas I come across more like . . . woman at C&A. What the hell am I going to do to compete with all this . . . insane wellness?

Then I start reading her latest inane-grin post. The hashtag is *#wellnessjourney* – urgh. Anyone who talks about figurative journeys needs to be shot. The only journey I'm interested in right now is to the corner shop to get some more red wine. But this opening salvo from Tara's post grabs my attention:

New job, new wellness goals.

Then she uses a couple of hashtags she hasn't mentioned yet: *#wellnessbootcamp*

What fresh hell is this? Then, this one catches my eye: *#rejuvenateyourself*

Now, I must admit, a bit of rejuvenation is something I could do with. I haven't felt rejuvenated in . . . well, maybe never. To be honest, even just looking at Tara's activities exhausts me. And I was already knackered tonight after work. I'm so bloody shattered all the time. Tired in my bones. Dragging myself through work like a zombie, collapsing on the sofa the minute I get home. No energy to cook let alone grocery shop, it's the same old routine of takeaway, wine and chocolate. If I wasn't stalking my frenemy, I'd be napping on the sofa by now. I read on, somewhat intrigued. After all, if I'm going to vanquish her, I need to know everything about her. And play her at her own game.

> *I'm starting on a new endeavour this week, friends. I've signed up for a wellness bootcamp called **January Rejuvenate**. (Click the link to find out more.) This great female-run start-up creates bespoke wellness journeys specifically aimed at women like us, women in their forties plus (though I've only one year left to claim that honour! Fifties here I come!).*

I knew it! Didn't I say she was forty-nine? Her fake welcome of her next decade makes me snort. We all know you're terrified, Tara. You'll be invisible before you know it. Anyway, back to the post. What the hell is this bootcamp thing?

> *Over the next four weeks, I'll be trying out a range of wellness treatments and therapies that are totally new to me. I can't wait to discover what wellness delights my new course will reward me with. And I'm keen to persuade you to join me on this new wellness adventure. Journeys are always best shared with friends! So, click here to find out more about the **January Rejuvenate** programme and when you join, we can chat about our wellness experiences here and share the wellness fun. Join me!*

If you'd told me this morning that I'd be googling a wellness bootcamp tonight, I'd have given you a breathalyser.

This was the last bloody thing I'd ever expect to be doing. But something tells me, I need to know what Tara is up to. I need information. Knowledge is power. And power is what I need over this interloper to my dream. If you can't beat 'em, join 'em, so they say. But I intend to join her, and then beat her. I click on the link.

It takes me to a sparkly website – literally, as it has little stars all over the page that are animated and glowing annoyingly – with a few paragraphs I can't be bothered to read about how two best friends founded the company after chatting in the playground on the school run blah blah blah. All right, yummy mummies, enough about you. Then, it goes on to the January Rejuvenate course itself. This is what I want to know about.

But then, my mobile rings and interrupts my snooping. Who the hell is ringing me at ten o'clock at night? The name pops up from WhatsApp. Shirley. Oh bloody hell, it's my sister. What on earth does she want? I consider letting it ring. And ring. After all, I haven't spoken to Shirley in a long time. We text sometimes, but hardly ever and mostly only about her two boys. I send them presents for their birthdays and Christmas, all the way to Wellington, New Zealand. That's not cheap, let me tell you. So, we exchange a text twice a year so I can see what my nephews are into these days, so the gifts aren't a complete waste of money. They're twelve and fourteen now, thus it won't be long until they just want cash.

Maybe Shirley's ringing about Mum. God, I haven't spoken to Mum in ages. She doesn't do texting. And we don't get on very well. She's seventy-seven this year and her health isn't great. Maybe something's happened, I suppose I must answer it.

'Hey, Shirl.'

'Lucy,' she says. My sister doesn't call me Lu. Or my mum. My dad used to. My nephews call me Auntie Lu, bless them. I do like Ned and Noah so much. They've got spirit and they get my sarcastic sense of humour unlike Shirley and Mum, who act like I'm a degenerate every time I swear. Dad used to swear like a trooper. Fucking hell, I miss him. It's been seven years and I still miss him every single day.

'What's up? Mum okay?'

'That's what I'm ringing about.'

'What's happened?' I feel a lurch of panic in my gut. I may not have seen Mum in person for six years but that doesn't mean I don't care.

'Mum's not well.'

'Tell me?'

'She had sort of a heart attack.'

'Is she okay?'

'I just told you, she's had a heart attack.'

'But what's her condition? Is she in hospital?'

'No, they took her in last night for monitoring, but she came home this morning. I'm keeping a close eye on her. Just thought you ought to know.'

'Is she there? Can I have a word with her?'

'She's sleeping. She needs her rest.'

'When you say, sort of a heart attack, what does that mean?'

'Well, they're not sure if it was a full-on heart attack. She had chest pain, racing pulse, pain in her arm, shallow breathing.'

'So, it might not've been a heart attack?'

'Would that be easier for you, if it wasn't?'

29

Shirley is an expert at crafting little digs at me about why I never moved out to New Zealand with them. After Dad's death, the heart was hollowed out of our family. We'd managed our differences because Dad always smoothed everything out. But once he was gone, we fell apart as a family. My mum and Shirl disappeared into their little clique and mourned together. I mourned alone. Then Shirl and her husband piped up that it was the perfect time to emigrate to New Zealand. It was a long-time plan of theirs anyway and Mum was up for it, as she was caught in the headlights after the loss of Dad and she just went along with anything Shirl said. And it was assumed I'd go with them, that we'd all emigrate and have a fresh start on the other side of the world, as far away from memories of Dad as possible. But I never wanted to. I didn't want to forget Dad. And my career was far too important to me. Shirl never forgave me, I don't think. And she seems to take pleasure in reminding me of that, every so often, or more like, every time we communicate. These little digs have the drip-drip effect of driving me nuts over time. She knows exactly how to press my buttons. I could have a stand-up row with her right now. She'd love that. She's always said how angry I can be. What she'll never admit is that her purse-lipped passive-aggressiveness is far angrier than I'll ever be. She just contains it. Dad used to say to me that letting out my rage is good for me, that Shirley and Mum kept it all inside where it festers. He taught me to swear with grace and howl at the moon. We used to go for walks in the High Weald, a national park of sorts, not far from here. And we'd find a quiet, beautiful place with no one around and raise our eyes to the sky and scream like banshees, let all the anger out. Then collapse in laughter. Extraordinary man, my dad.

I let out a sigh. 'Shirl, don't start, please.'

'I'm not starting. I'm just run ragged with this lot. I'm exhausted. Looking after the kids, and Mum. It's a huge responsibility. I'm stuck in the middle of two generations who need me twenty-four-seven. You couldn't understand familial responsibility, as you have no responsibilities, Lucy. You never have.'

I could rise to that, but I don't bother. I don't want to fall out with my sister. Her voice still has a bit of the Kentish twang, but after six years in New Zealand, it's morphed into an amalgam of the two which makes her feel increasingly foreign to me. They're in Wellington, where Shirley's husband Ray works as a dentist and she is a stay-at-home mum and carer to our mother who lives with them – though the truth is that, until this heart attack scare, whatever Shirley says, Mum doesn't need that much caring for. She's mobile, she's compos mentis and she can easily get the bus into town. True, she has type two diabetes and sometimes gets some nasty skin rashes, but other than that, she's not too bad for her age. But according to Shirl, our mum is at death's door constantly.

I sigh and try conciliation instead of the knee-jerk reaction I could give. 'Shirl, I love you all. You know I do. I love your boys. I always send presents for them. I love the memes Ned sends me.'

'Ned sends you what?'

'Memes. On Instagram. They're hilarious! He's got Dad's sense of humour down to a tee.'

'I don't understand memes. Neither does Mum. Who are

the people in the pictures anyway? What are they talking about? Stupid things.'

'Well, your kid loves them. Maybe you should get him to send you some.'

Shirley humphs and says, 'I don't need him to text me. I'm here. With him. For him. Same as I am for Mum. Same as you'd be, if you'd not been so career-mad and come with us. It's wrong, me being the one who has to look after everyone. You get to live there scot-free. Free as a bird.'

This old chestnut. The rage is coming off her in waves. I can feel it viscerally down the phone.

'I'm sorry you're drowning in it right now,' I say. 'I truly am. But you are the one that decided to move away. That was your choice, Shirl. Yours and Mum's. You wanted to go to the ends of the earth after we . . . after we lost Dad. But I didn't want that. I visit his grave regularly. I tidy it up and leave flowers. I have a chat with him.'

'No point conversing with the dead when the living are here. You should be here, in the land of the living, where you're needed. It's not as if you've got anything to stay for over there. No husband, no children. Just your ridiculous loyalty to your job. You should be here, where Mum needs you. And you could take the pressure off me. I know you think Mum is okay, because you're thinking of the mum you knew six years ago. But she's in decline. She's gone downhill. Dad doesn't need you to visit his grave. He's dead and gone for seven years now.'

Now it's my turn to feel the rage swell in me. I can't bear it when Shirl slags off our dad. They never got on well. She never understood him. Neither did Mum, not really. Maybe she did when they met, but as they got older, she just found him annoying. They both did, Shirl and Mum, in their little coterie. The effort to not let rip down the phone and scream at her is painful.

'Shirl, let's not do this right now. I've had a shitty day. Trouble at work. And I'm shattered.'

'Well, I'll leave you to it. I've got to go. I'm just doing my duty, letting you know. I've no idea if you wanted to hear about it or not. But I want to do the right thing.'

'I know you do. And of course I want to know.'

There's a pronounced silence. Then, Shirl says, with an air of defeat, 'I know you do too.'

She can't keep up her rage for long. We still love each other, my sister and I, underneath all the angst.

'All right, Shirl. Keep me posted. Send Mum my love. And the boys and Ray. And love to you too.'

Shirley hangs up, without even saying goodbye. How did it come to this? Sure, we'd fall out sometimes when we were younger, like all siblings do. But since I said no to emigrating with them, I've become the enemy, somehow. They could not fathom why I didn't want to come. Especially once Martin had left me. It was utterly confounding to both Mum and Shirley why I'd want to stay here alone, when they were all moving to beautiful New Zealand. The High Weald is beautiful too, I told them. And Dad was still here. In the ground, yes. But still here. They thought I was mad. They thought I'd change my mind. They don't understand me. They don't get how important my job is to me, how I've worked my arse off for thirty years to get where I am. And the top job, the one I want more than anything, was just out of reach. But I was sure, if I stuck it out, if I did my best and waited, eventually, finally, the COO post would come and it'd be mine.

Or so I thought. For now, Tara bloody Harryman and her perfect life and her power hairdo stand in my way. And if I don't get this promotion, everything I've stood my ground for with my family in the last six years will mean nothing. I simply must beat this usurper to the prize. And I can see I have my work cut out for me, with wellness guru of the year here. At least I know a bit more about her now. I get myself to bed, as that conversation with Shirl has really done me in. I'm off for a good night's sleep, before the fight-back begins at 9am tomorrow with a meeting between me, Derek and Tara. But I'll be going armed this time. Let battle commence.

Chapter 4

The next day, Tara has a smart trouser suit on, again with impressively tall heels. I don't know how she doesn't get bunions with those things. Or plantar fasciitis. Maybe she does. Maybe she suffers for her perfect corporate image. Urgh, I need to stop staring at her. She'll think I'm a psychopath. But the truth is, I'm jealous of her. She looks great for her age. I look at least my age, if not older. And there's only four years between us. But I remind myself that it's our corporate skills that will get us this job, not our skincare routine. That's what I keep telling myself, anyway.

Derek is rambling on about Tara's new role as director of legal services and we're discussing legislation that's coming into the insurance sector and other such illuminating subjects, while Tara drinks ionised water. I have no idea what ionised water is. But that's what it says on the bottle she pours from into an office glass. There are plenty of water coolers here to choose from, but Tara brings in her own ionised water from home.

In a quick break from proceedings, while Derek answers his mobile briefly, I ask Tara, 'What is ionised water?'

'Oh, it's so good!' she enthuses. 'It's basically alkaline water. Really good for your pH. Really good for your gut too. And significantly decreases your risk of cancer.'

Cancer-beating water? What a load of bollocks. My God, this woman is a walking cliché of wellness. Does she really think ionised water is going to save her life? Cancer doesn't give a damn if you drink holy water from a sacred well on Mount Olympus. It'll get you anyway. I bet her dumb water costs a fortune. I bet all this wellness bullshit costs an arm and a leg. Then, as if I summoned it, Derek comes off his phone and immediately mentions wellness. I didn't know he'd ever heard the word before.

'Tara has been telling me all about workplace wellness,' says Derek enthusiastically.

'We have a policy for that, as I'm sure you're aware,' I say to Derek. Tara may be a fancy shmancy legal adviser, but I'm director of HR and I'm the one in charge of staff welfare, and wellness, if we must use that word.

'Of course, but from what Tara says I think there's far more to it. Isn't that right, Tara?'

'Yes, Derek. And I know, Lucy, that Beane & Co have a robust policy in place for staff wellness. However, I do think there's more we can do.'

She flourishes a copy of our workplace wellness policy – that I wrote – that she happens to have printed out beforehand. *Here's one I prepared earlier*, as they used to say on *Blue Peter*.

Tara adds, 'It's very well written and conceived, of course, Lucy. But I do think there's scope here for more. There is a plethora of wellness courses out there we could arrange for our staff. Really get them thinking about their physical and mental wellness, and its effect on their productivity. There's plenty of recent scientific research supporting this.'

'Scientific research, yes,' says Derek, nodding like a parakeet who doesn't understand a bloody word. Tara's clearly learnt quickly how to impress Derek.

'For example,' she goes on, 'I'm just about to start a wellness bootcamp this month.'

Oh God, here we go. Yes, I know all about it, Tara. I stalked your socials last night. But I can't let her know that, obviously.

'Bootcamp?' says Derek, all perked up. 'I like the sound of that! Put our staff through their paces!'

Tara laughs, like little bells tinkling or crystalline water tumbling over rocks. Even her laugh is perfect.

'Not at all, Derek. These are meant to improve you, mind, body and soul.'

Speaking in hashtags, Tara? How unoriginal.

'It's a four-week course called January Rejuvenate, where participants choose four wellness treatments to enlighten them about their mental and physical condition, so that they can then go on to perfect their own wellness routines, streamlining their bodies and minds into their purest forms, with the richest potential and prime optimisation. We owe it to ourselves to be the best version of ourselves that we can possibly be. Don't you think, Derek?'

Gah, the bullshit jargon! The self-righteousness! The rage is boiling in me now and I'm about to blow. But I'm bloody glad now I did stalk this damn woman last night. Knowledge is power, as I said.

'Gosh!' cries Derek. 'That does sound impressive. I don't suppose you know anything about this, do you, Lucia? Doesn't sound like your bag at all! Have you heard of this January bootcamp thingy?'

'Heard of it?' I say, with a smug smile. 'I've signed up for it already.'

What . . . what did I just say? What words leapt out of my mouth before I had the chance to kill them at the source?

'You've signed up for the January Rejuvenate course?' says Tara, eyeing me suspiciously. I can tell she wasn't expecting that in a million years. And I've gone and done it now. There's no going back.

'Absolutely. The one by that local company, a super start-up run by two women.'

'Yes, yes, I know,' says Tara. Ha! She's really rattled now. 'Wow, so, you're doing it too? What a coincidence.'

She's probably guessed I stalked her. But she can't prove it. And Derek doesn't have a clue.

'Jolly good!' says Derek. 'You two are on the same page already. That's marvellous. Listen, Lucia, that gives me an idea. We've got the staff conference coming up in three months and, of course, it'll be my last one ever. I really want to go out with a bang, to secure my legacy and I think workplace wellness is the thing for it. I want my staff to know how much I care about them, to remind them how much I've *always* cared about them. Make them recall me fondly as time goes by, once I'm retired from this place. I say we make workplace wellness the theme of the conference and, Lucia, your annual speech should be about this very thing. You're doing that wellness bootcamp thing, so you can report back about it all in your speech and give us all a boost. Capital idea! Well done, Tara, and Lucia. I have good vibrations about all this stuff, you two, all this wellness stuff. Jolly good. And I'm certain Nick will be very impressed with the two of you and this initiative, very impressed.'

And so, my fate is sealed. Not only have I lied about signing up for some godawful bullshit I'd never do willingly in a million years, I've also got to make a speech about it and organise the whole staff conference around the subject of wellness, a subject I think is the biggest load of bollocks there is. What the hell have I landed myself in? Tara is looking at me with renewed interest. I'm trying to discern her expression. There's a little smile there, that might be smugness – I'm sure she's twigged that I lied about having signed up for the course – but there's also a smidgeon of respect there. Her face seems to be saying, 'Game on.'

The rest of the day is stuffed with meetings and paperwork, and I'm delighted to leave at five. I need to rush down to town to see my bestie Jacqui at the cinema. We always meet a couple of hours before the film so we can have a good gossip first. And have I got some gossip for her.

When I arrive in the car park, I'm about to text Jacqui to say I'm here in the car park, because I hate going in anywhere and waiting alone, people staring at me, thinking I'm weird because I'm on my own. But instead I find a text from my sister Shirley.

It wasn't a heart attack.

Oh. Okay. That's typical Shirl. No soft openers or emojis.

Hey Shirl. That's good news, right?

Yes. It turns out she has a prolapsed disc in her neck causing referred pain in her arm. They've started her on painkillers and physio. The painkillers are helping. The other symptoms were probably an anxiety attack.

What's Mum anxious about?

Everything. You'd know if you were here.

Urgh, here we go again. I can't be getting into all that now.

But she's feeling better now, yeah?

Yes, she's doing well. She's complaining that she's bored in bed and hates NZ daytime TV, even though we have all the streaming services but Mum hates those too and won't use them. Apparently it's unnatural to have too much choice on television, as 'the channels know best what we ought to watch'.

Sounds like typical Mum, i.e. utterly fake logic. But I don't have time right now to discuss all of Mum's annoying habits.

Glad she's ok. But I'm rushing off now as going to meet a friend at the cinema, sorry.

We can't have you missing your film.

Everything Shirl says always sounds like a threat.

Thanks and please send Mum my love and tell her not to be anxious. She lives in beautiful New Zealand after all!

Don't be ridiculous.

Catch you later, Shirl

No reply. And I'm off. I'm so happy to be putting that conversation and all its implications away in my handbag and trotting inside to see Jacqui.

I'm so grateful I have Jacqui in my life. She's the only one who understands me, truly *gets* me, you know? I don't have to try with her, I don't have to tidy up my house before she shows up, I don't have to pretend to be happy or wear make-up or anything. We became friends in the third year at school, when we were both thirteen. Blimey, that's forty years ago! Forty! We're so old now. I need to remind her we should celebrate our forty-year anniversary. She was the new girl who had just arrived at the girls' grammar I was at because her parents had split up and she'd had to move halfway across the country. I was sick and tired of the girls in my class, so petty and immature. I liked her from day one. She had crimped hair which looked the quintessence of cool. She was mad about writing, always carrying a little notebook and tiny pencil around with her. She collected pencils, special ones, kept in a shoebox. I collected erasers, also kept in a shoebox. It was meant to be. Friends for life.

And there she is, sitting at the cinema bar on a tall stool, sipping a cocktail with an umbrella in it. She's got her long, shaggy blonde hair dragged into a side ponytail that drapes over her shoulder and she's wearing jeans and a vintage mustard-yellow seventies blouse she no doubt found in a second-hand store. Effortlessly stylish is Jacqui, always has been. I look like an M&S mannequin from the business section. But I don't care and neither does Jacqui. None of that matters with your bestie. She looks up from her phone and sees me approach.

'Lu!' she cries and two teen lads on a leather sofa beneath an enormous cheese plant jump at the sound, as Jacqui's voice is so bloody loud.

'Jac!' I shout, alarming the boys again, as they nurse their Cokes and start muttering and smirking. But we don't give a shit.

We throw our arms around each other and she nearly falls off the stool and we laugh.

'Cocktails at 5.15pm! What a grand idea. Shame I've got the car.'

'It really is a grand idea,' says Jacqui. 'I was working from home today and it was shit, so I walked here early. Time for a negroni, I decided. Shit day yourself?'

'So shit. Plus my mum's ill.'

'What's up?'

I tell her about it all. 'Mum sounds absolutely back to normal now. That is, infuriating as ever. Anyway, how are you? How's work? How're the kids, how's Barna?'

'He's over in Hungary visiting his mum. He actually gets on with his mum, unlike you and me. He *actually wants* to go and see her! How bizarre is that?!'

'Weirdo,' I say.

I'm only joking, though. Jacqui's husband Barna is not a weirdo at all. He's ace. He runs his own cleaning business and charms all his customers, with his lovely accent and his bad jokes. They're a smashing couple, Jac and Barna. They met in a local club in their thirties, drunk as skunks. They

42

were married within six months. A great love story. And well deserved. They have three gorgeous kids who all call me Auntie Lu, just like my real nephews. I'm a brilliant aunt, real and honorary, I must say. Made for it. I find I can easily love kids, when they're someone else's. I know Jacqui isn't having the easiest time with them though, at the moment, specifically her eldest son, Harvey, who's fifteen and going through some medical issues. Jacqui's really worried about him.

We talk about Harvey and we talk about her girls, Freya, twelve, and Holly, nine. She's such a brilliant mum, intimately involved in every aspect of their lives. And still managing to work full-time as a journalist at the *Kent Today* newspaper, up in Maidstone, nearly an hour's commute during rush hour. I take my hat off to her. I've no kids and a tiny commute and I'm stressed out. I don't know how she does it.

'I'm sick and tired of work,' Jacqui sighs.

'Same old problem with your useless twat of a boss?'

'Yup. The stories he lets me work on are rubbish. Last week, I'm sure you saw my illustrious byline on the story of the week: Dog Dirt on Slide.'

I burst out laughing.

'Stop laughing!' says Jacqui, laughing too.

'Some great alliteration there!' I say. 'You did your best getting those two Ds in and avoiding the word "shit".'

'I did, didn't I! But it's not exactly going to get me Journalist of the Year, is it?'

She looks glum and, though we often have a good chuckle about the stories she has foisted on her, it gets her down.

'I know you've felt this way for a couple of years now,

since this new boss idiot came along. Can you try talking to him about it again?'

Jacqui shakes her head. 'He's cloth-eared, believe me. Anyway, I don't want to talk about work.' She sighs. 'It depresses me. How's work for you after all the drama of Derek's retirement announcement? How's Tara Bitchface?'

'Oh my God!' I cry. 'This is the gossip I have for you. I've totally royally fucked up and landed myself in it.'

'What? What?!' Jacqui says, hopping up and down on her backside and taking another slurp of her negroni.

'I've inadvertently signed up for a four-week wellness bootcamp, by accident.'

Jacqui bursts out laughing. 'A wellness what? A fucking WHAT? And by accident?!'

She's giggling madly. I'm looking at her with my eyebrows raised and pursed lips, waiting for her hilarity to subside, though I'm loving it. I knew this would make her piss herself. However shitty my news might be, it's always worth it to make Jacqui laugh. She loves my rage-filled rants about work.

'Explain everything!' she demands. So, I tell her the whole sorry tale.

'Basically I tried to impress my boss and ended up lying and dropping myself in a world of shit. Wellness bootcamp! Me? Fuck my life.'

'Oh, this is delicious!' laughs Jacqui, uncontrollably.

'Thanks for the schadenfreude,' I mutter, but I can't help but laugh too. The whole situation is ridiculous.

'You're welcome! What does it involve? What do you have to do?'

'I've no idea. Probably just drinking smoothies and power walking.'

'You mean, you haven't checked it out properly?'

'Oh God, you know what? I haven't even googled it myself since last night, because my sister interrupted. I've no bloody idea what I'm supposed to have signed up for. Let's have a look.'

'What's it called? I'm googling it!'

Jacqui finds it and scrolls down to the description. She reads it aloud.

'Okay, here we go. It says, "In our January Rejuvenate Wellness Bootcamp, we gift you four sessions of wellness that will transform your being. Choose from a selection of groundbreaking therapies that will root you in a holistic treatment plan, where you can take exactly what is requisite for your own selfhood from respected modalities within our gamechanger community of wellness gurus. Don't forget though, you are your own guru, so harness your inner power through connectedness and open up new pathways to wholeness."'

'What in God's name are these people talking about?!' I cry.

'It's buzzword heaven! Jesus Christ, this is cliché gold. We've hit the mother lode!'

'Seriously, though, I don't understand a word.'

'You're not supposed to. Blind you with pseudo-science, that's the game. I need another negroni for this,' she says, swigging back the last of it, then calling over the barman. Jacqui lives in walking distance of the cinema and I don't, but, bloody hell, I could do with a cocktail right now. Something to dilute all this bullshit.

'What the hell have I signed up for? What are the choices anyway?'

We have a look at the list. There are eight to choose from, four to pick. The list is as follows:

- The Ice Experience
- Vigour Surge Formula
- Aura Imaging
- Vitality Oils Workshop
- Magno Suppository Healing
- Fossil Therapy
- Clarity with Clio
- Quantum Brain Retune

After reading that lot, Jacqui literally falls off her stool crying with laughter (plus I think the negronis on an empty stomach don't help). The barman comes round to help her up which makes us laugh even more.

'How are you going to choose from that lot of absolute wank?' Jacqui is saying, between bouts of uncontrollable giggles. 'Just don't let them shove anything up your arse!'

'Never! Never!' I cry. 'What the fuck am I going to do?!' Then, a sharp fear comes over me. I haven't even looked at the price. 'Hang on, how much is all this nonsense going to cost me?'

Once Jacqui is safely back on her stool, and been given a pint of water and a bag of crisps by the sensible barman, I start tapping my way round the site to try to find the price list. Finally, I find it ensconced in a webpage rabbit-hole so deep, I wouldn't be surprised to see Alice in Wonderland down there with me.

'SIX HUNDRED QUID?'

Jacqui hoots.

I say, hopelessly, 'What the hell am I doing to do?'

'You're gonna do it, chick. Show your commitment to wellness to impress the bossmen. And entertain me with regular gory debriefs. I need a laugh. Even if it's at your expense.'

'Well, I'm committed to the expense of at least six hundred quid now, for fuck's sake. God, I'm an idiot.'

'Yeah, you are,' laughs Jackie. 'But if it gets you your dream job, then it'll be worth it, eh?'

I picture in my mind's eye my new role as COO, working on strategy and vision with our new CEO and looking down on Tara in her measly director's role and never having to deal with the likes of minions like loudmouth Lorraine from Accounts or bolshy Barry from Sales ever again. That would be absolute heaven on earth. Maybe I can do this wellness thing. Maybe I can ace it and impress the hell out of Nick Bridges.

'Oh shit, what's the time?' Jacqui says.

'Oh yeah, we were gassing so much. We need to get our tickets. What are we seeing at the flicks again?'

'We couldn't decide. Some family drama or some horror thing.'

'Horror thing,' I say. 'I can't be arsed with family tonight.'

Chapter 5

I'm forced to sign up for the damned January Rejuvenate, now I've bragged I've already signed up, which I'm pretty sure Tara knows was a lie but Derek doesn't seem to have twigged a thing. Nick Bridges popped in again the day after the cinema and Derek was telling him all about our new wellness policies taking shape and that Tara and *Lucia* (urgh) were doing all the research now and would present the new policy at the staff conference in a few weeks' time. Nick looked suitably impressed and said it was 'right on the money of windows of change', whatever the fuck that means.

I'm on the sofa again with a nice little slurp of Tempranillo and it's time to book my four sessions. I've had a look at the list and the explanations of each, which still don't make much sense, but – as Jacqui said – anything up my arse is out of the question, so that ticks off Magno Suppository Healing (which apparently is a fancy name for colonic irrigation somehow involving magnets? Don't ask me how . . .). The other ones I chuck out are as follows:

Vigour Surge Formula – this involves channelling photons from the sun's rays into the soles of your feet via the power of thought, which causes an energy surge through your system to kill off all bad bacteria. I mean . . . just . . . fuck off.

Aura Imaging – we would spend an hour using wax crayons to draw each other's auras, then compare and contrast. Crayolas are used specifically to provide a channel for our inner child to speak through our auras. If I wanted to spend significant amounts of money on colouring in, I'd buy Caran D'Ache, thanks very much, and they *still* wouldn't be as expensive as this crap.

Quantum Brain Retune – something to do with wearing sunglasses and listening to white noise while breathing in shallow pulses and releasing toxins from . . . oh, I can't even be bothered to finish explaining it to you. It's not happening. No way, no how.

The remaining four all sound relatively harmless but still pretty vague. Okay, so my first session will be the Ice Experience. I'm thinking ice baths? It doesn't explain much, just that it will change my life. Oh, good. And to bring a swimming costume. Warm towels and bathrobe provided. I book it in for this Friday evening and spend the rest of the week at work casually dropping it into conversation whenever Tara is around, how much I'm looking forward to it and can't wait to learn new things to optimise my wellness routines and all that bollocks. Tara keeps pretty schtum about it. She doesn't give anything away, that one. Keeps herself to herself, except with Derek and Nick. It's a clever tactic because she's an unknown quantity – and it's working . . . because I'm more fascinated by her than ever. Who is she, really? Does she want the COO job as much as I do? I think she does as she's working overtime on sucking up to the CEOs. Every time I try to make conversation with her, she keeps it short and polite, then snaps it off as quickly as possible. I reckon she knows knowledge is power too. Oh well, sod her. I just need to get through this next month and the four stupid wellness sessions and present some rubbish about it at the staff conference and then I reckon I'm home and dry.

Friday night rolls around and I arrive at a village about halfway between here and Tonbridge called Bidborough. I park up where the satnav takes me, outside a house down a leafy lane. I have another look at the confirmation email which I'd only briefly scanned before setting off and realise that the name of the practitioner tonight is Boudicca. Of course she's called Boudicca. You can't be called Sharon and be a wellness practitioner. You have to have something outlandish, don't you? I wonder if it actually says Boudicca on her birth certificate. Does it, Boudicca, eh? I might ask her. Anyway, I go up to the front door and there's the classic hippy symbol of the 'green man' on her door knocker. Of course there is. I'm expecting the overpowering fug of joss stick smoke. I knock and wait. There comes a little shout from the side of the house and I wander round there to find a short woman with a cloud of gorgeous white curly hair and what Jacqui and I used to call a hippy skirt on.

'Lucy Cooper, is it?' she says, with a lovely smile and a deep Kentish accent. I like her already.

'That's me,' I say and she invites me in through the side entrance, into a small waiting room with a cubicle in the corner.

'Welcome, welcome, Lucy Cooper,' she says. 'Your name is ever so mellifluous, has anyone ever told you that?'

'No.' I've been in a bad mood all day in anticipation of this forced fun, but she's so nice about it all that I feel churlish being rude, so I make an effort. 'But thank you.'

'Yes, yes, it sounds like water trickling through a dark tunnel. Luuuuucy Coooooooper. Trickle trickle!'

Now I want to go for a pee.

Boudicca adds, 'Now, shall we begin?'

'Yes please,' I say, because I want to get it over with as swiftly as possible. She instructs me to go into the changing cubicle in the corner of the waiting room and put on my bathing costume and one of the towel robes hanging in there. She says there's a range of sizes. Good, because I'll be choosing the biggest one so I can hide in it. I'm starting to regret selecting this session, since I hate showing my body to anyone, to be honest. But at least nothing will get shoved up my backside. I go into the cubicle grateful for that at least. Boudicca calls out that I should come through into the therapy room when I'm ready.

On the wall in the cubicle is a poster of a bumble bee with the immortal legend above, *What will be, will be.* Thanks, bee, but what the fuck do you know about philosophy anyway? I fold up my clothes on the little stool in there – carefully ensuring my knickers and bra are hidden beneath my folded polo neck jumper, of course. I mean, even when I'm having a smear test and the nurse is about to see every damn thing, I still fold up my knickers so they can't be seen.

I come out and see the door to the next room and go through it. The therapy room itself is larger and decorated sparsely with everything painted white and silky flowers with little lights in them draped from corner to corner against the pure white walls. There's a countertop on one wall with two stools beside it and an under-counter fridge. On another wall is a large white cupboard which is plugged in. Maybe that's where she warms the towels promised in the blurb. Near the far wall is a bathtub, one of those nice old-fashioned free-standing clawfoot baths. I've always wanted one of those. I can just see from here that it's filled with water with a load of ice cubes piled up in there. I'm assuming I'm supposed to go and get in it for a few seconds and get out and then our session is done. That's what I'm hoping anyway. But no, we have to stretch it out to an hour to get my money's worth, I suppose. Boudicca starts with an introduction to our session.

'Before beginning the Ice Experience, we must prepare our body. It'd be quite a shock to the system if you just jumped in icy cold water with no warning. Our brain knows we're about to do it, but our body is always playing catch-up, so we need to help it on its way. Please disrobe, placing your robe on the countertop and then we will be doing some exercises to prepare your body.'

I do so, feeling self-conscious, but I did at least pick a bathing costume with a little skirt and plenty of coverage at the neckline, so as much of myself is covered up as possible. I stand opposite Boudicca on the white tiled floor (which is a bit chilly on the feet) and she tells me to follow her lead. She starts with a couple of movements familiar to me from yoga, which I never did but my ex, Martin, used to do in the living room sometimes. I'm getting a bit puffed just doing these gentle stretches. I don't do anything to move my body around these days. Perhaps I ought to take up yoga. Boudicca and I do a few more movements that she calls sun salutations, then we stand up and Boudicca places her hands on her hips and so do I.

'Now that we're a little warmed up,' she says, 'we must access the universal divine feminine power through the following movements. This is what will keep you safe in the icy water.'

Okay . . . She starts by swaying her hips from side to side, moving them in a circle. Then we're thrusting our hips forward in increasingly jerky movements, which feels weird and looks even weirder. This goes on for far longer than I'm sure is necessary. You're really dragging this out, aren't you, Boudicca? How on earth this accesses the universal divine feminine power is anyone's guess. Then, at last, we're ready for me to take the plunge, literally. We go over to the bath. I stand beside it, feeling a bit nervy. I really don't want to sit in an ice bath. I mean it's going to be . . . really cold! Urgh, best get it over with.

'Jump in!' says Boudicca, grinning.

'Well, okay, but if I jump, won't the water go everywhere?'

'Don't fret about that. It's a tiled floor with a slight slope and a drain over there. It's designed to take the water.'

I don't care, I'm still not going to jump in a bath. I can see myself slipping and cracking my head open. So, I step in gingerly and the cold is immediate and shocking.

'Oh!' I cry and immediately pull out my foot.

'No, no, go back in. Let it envelop you. You must follow through. You must step in and then sit down, submerge yourself up to your neck in the iced water. You'll then stay in for forty-five seconds, that is all. You can do it, Lucy! I have the upmost faith in you.'

It's the *utmost* faith, actually, Boudicca. But this is no time for pedantry. I've got two feet in now and I want to go home. It's really bloody cold. I mean, obviously. But it's like knives. Maybe I have ultra-sensitive skin. I do get weird rashes unreasonably often, like Mum does. The sooner I sit down

53

and get this over with, the sooner I can go home. So I sit down with a bump and, as I predicted, almost slip, and as a result, slide all the way under the water, soaking my hair and coming up spluttering. God, this is horrible. The cold is horrible. I want to get out! Boudicca is counting up to forty-five now and every second seems to stretch on for an aeon. Christ, I'm pathetic, aren't I? I can't even stand less than a minute in something uncomfortable? Think of the job! Think of the kudos! Think of anything but a million little knives stabbing your skin all over. While she's counting, Boudicca puts down a bathmat for me, then fetches a towel from the cupboard and holds it out because FINALLY the task is over and I get up as quickly as I can without hazard, grasp onto the side of the bath and step out onto the mat. Immediately she wraps the huge, warm towel around me and I've never wanted a warm towel more (in fact, I've never had a warm towel, in my life. I never had one of those burns-unit-style bathroom towel heater thingies, though I always kind of wanted one).

Boudicca then passes me my towelling robe as well and I put that on over the top. Ah, heaven.

'How was it?' she asks, smiling.

'Awful! I hated it!'

'How do you feel now?'

'So much better.'

'Better than when you were in the bath, or better than you were before you came here tonight?'

Now, that makes me think. On the way here, I was feeling really tired and fed up. Really achy from a long week at work. In short, I was feeling crap. And now . . . ?

'Well, actually . . . I am feeling good. I feel . . . pretty great, to be honest. That's not a word I use very often.'

Boudicca looks delighted. Oh shit, did I just . . . enjoy a wellness activity? Not enjoy, as such, but I feel like I have got something out of it.

'Good! Now then, the next stage is over here. Please be seated at the bar.'

By bar, she means the countertop with a student-bedsit-sized fridge underneath it. She takes from it a large jug of pinky-purple liquid, which she pours into a tall glass and places before me.

'You need to drink all of this, every drop.'

'What is it . . . ?' I say, eyeing up its weird colour.

'It's a detox cleanse which you'll need now the cold water has surfaced all of the toxins in your body. This will cleanse you of those toxins.'

'What's in it?'

'This is my own secret recipe which I only share with my clients in private sessions, because modern medicine and Big Pharma don't want you to know the truth.'

'What truth?'

'How sick the world is making you. These natural ingredients create a holistic approach to your inner wellness, complementing the healing power of the ice bath. This secret recipe came to me from my spirit guide.'

Uh-oh, and we were doing so well.

'Your what?'

'My spirit guide shows me how to help others. He gave me the recipe for this juice cleanse.'

Okay then . . . so when I'm dead, I'll be spending my ghostly time sending shit recipes back to the earthly realm? Is that all the afterlife has to offer?!

'Well, Boudicca, I'm sorry but I've made it a kind of life

rule never to drink something when I don't know what's in it. Sorry.'

'I see you have a cautious spirit, my dear, but I understand. We have allergens to consider even though you didn't mention anything on your booking form, very well. The secret recipe handed down to me by my spirit guide is a pint of radicchio juice with cayenne pepper and a quarter teaspoon of Mānuka honey. All of these ingredients promote oxygen in the blood, as well as remove toxins.'

'But isn't that what our liver and kidneys are doing, all the time? Detoxing our body, I mean? Isn't that literally their job?'

'Oh, no,' says Boudicca, shaking her head which makes her fluffy white hair bob from side to side. 'That's not detoxing enough. There are invisible toxins you can't see and your organs don't know about. Drink up.'

My organs don't know about . . . ? Sounds like her reasoning behind all of these rituals is distinctly suspect. Well, I've got a pretty cast-iron stomach. Can't remember the last time I had the shits. So I take a swig of it.

Jeez Louise, the juice tastes like dirty dishwater steeped in a spicy kind of sadness.

'Drink it all down!' Boudicca cries loudly, which nearly makes me choke on it.

I really don't want to. I tell her I have a medical condition which means I can't drink too much liquid at any one time. Then she's annoyed at me for not mentioning that when I booked, so she looks at me suspiciously and I'm looking at her suspiciously too. Then she breaks the stand-off by leaving to fetch more ice to heave into the tub and we do some more weird hip thrusting, before I'm back in the tub. This happens three more times – five in total. By the end, I'm exhausted. I've done bugger all but I feel like I've been swimming lengths for an hour.

I'm glad when it's over. Boudicca extols the virtues of ice baths and – the next best thing apparently – taking a cold shower every morning and every night. She asks me to promise I'll do it.

'I promise I will,' I lie.

'Excellent!' she says. 'It's very good for the skin of us older ladies. Which reminds me, I have a special offer on just now, exclusively for my private clients. My business partner, Sandy, runs a clinic next door in salmon sperm facials. Fully qualified, is Sandy. Only £400. Until the end of January. Grab it now, while you can.'

I recoil in disgust. Salmon . . . what? Salmon SPERM FACIAL??? Fuck no.

'Not today, thank you,' I say and retreat to the changing cubicle.

Once I'm changed, I shake Boudicca's hand and thank her for the experience.

'Come again soon!' she says, as she shows me out. 'Don't forget, contact with ice water cures all diseases or at least many, many diseases. It's been proven by lots and lots of anecdotal evidence.'

Anecdotal evidence? Well, that proves it then. May as well book the salmon jizz while I'm at it. Which makes me wonder, what the hell are they doing to those poor fish? Does it happen in the appointment? Does her friend Sandy hoist a salmon out of a tank and . . . pleasure it? The mind boggles.

I wave at Boudicca as I get into my car, then get the hell out of there. I go over the events of the last hour during my drive home. There was so much to take the piss out of, I don't know where to start. I can't wait to tell Jacqui later about this nonsense. Spirit guides? Unknowing organs? Purple lettuce juice? But the ice bath thing . . . I must admit, it felt good afterwards. I did feel invigorated. Maybe it's just the contrast between the misery of being sat in ice and the warm towel after. Maybe that's all it was. But it does make me wonder if a cold shower now and again wouldn't do any harm . . . maybe, behind all the gumph, there is some good to be found in this wellness stuff.

Once I'm home, I message Jacqui and tell her all about it. Jacqui texts back:

You not heard of Salmon Sperm Facials? One of the Kardashians has those. It's on YouTube I think.

I reply:

Please tell me there's not a video of someone wanking off a fish all over a Kardashian's face.

Also . . . send me a link. (For a friend.)

Chapter 6

Of course, I don't share my true thoughts about Boudicca and her mauve juice cleanse and recipe-sending spirit healer at work. But I do boast about it to Derek after a meeting in the conference room this week, within Tara's earshot, saying how invigorating the ice bath was and how I've been having cold showers ever since as they've improved my circulation and given me so much more energy (lies, lies and more lies).

Derek laughs and says, 'In my day, cold showers meant something a bit different! You'd only have one if, you know, you needed to . . . calm down *below*, if you know what I mean!'

He's just about modern enough to know not to go into detail on that one and instead turns away, chuckling, and leaves the room. Tara, standing behind him, involuntarily grimaces at his crass joke. That makes me smile. Maybe she finds Derek insufferable too. Maybe we've got something in common after all.

I turn to Tara and say, 'Have you done the Ice Experience yet? I highly recommend it, if not.'

'I didn't choose that one, no,' says Tara. 'I already take cold showers every morning anyway.'

Urgh. Of course she does. My brief feeling of solidarity with her vanishes.

'I've got Vitality Oils Workshop next, whatever that means. I hope it's not rubbing oils all over me. Always sounds a bit greasy. Which sessions have you done so far, then?' I ask. I must keep up with her, so I need to know what she's up to.

'Clarity with Clio.'

'How was it?'

She pauses for a moment, then says, 'Life-changing.'

I can tell she really means it. I've signed up for that one too.

'In what way? I'm doing that one too. It's last on my list.'

'You'll see,' she says and shrugs her shoulders. And there's a hint of a smile there.

Look, I know she's my rival, but that doesn't mean we have to hate each other, does it? I mean, I do hate her, don't get me wrong. And talking to her is like pulling teeth. I want to say to her, *for God's sake, Tara, throw me a bone here*! But also, I can't deny I am intrigued by her. I'm about to say something about how I'm looking forward to it, or other pleasantries, when she suddenly says something else.

'Do you like being called Lucia?'

'No, I bloody don't,' I say.

She nods emphatically and purses her lips, you know that way people do when they suspect something that's then confirmed.

Then, she just walks off, out of the room. See what I mean about intriguing? I'm wondering, once all this competition bullshit is over, whether Tara and I might even be friends one day, who knows? But . . . only if I win, obviously.

So, this week's Friday adventure is as follows: the Vitality Oils Workshop with Steve. (Steve? That's a deadly dull name. Like he's not even trying. Not exactly Boudicca, is it. Try harder, Steve!)

This one's on the outskirts of Tunbridge Wells, in a little industrial estate alongside a soft play centre and a psychoanalyst. Just imagine if all three joined forces. Now that's the kind of therapy I could get behind. So, there's a general front door and I ring and a receptionist lets me in and directs me down this long corridor to room 27 at the end. This building looks like a prefab that might blow over in a stiff breeze. I reach number 27 and knock on the door and a voice says, 'Come in!' with enthusiasm. I try the handle and the whole door frame rattles and I'm even more convinced this is a theatre set that'll collapse if I touch anything. I push the door inwards and the stink of various sickly-sweet odours floods out as if imprisoned in there, desperate to escape.

Inside the room, it's pretty dim and the first thing I see is a tall water feature thing with bubbles going up and down a tube, also with little plastic fish bobbing about. At least, I hope they're plastic, as I don't have my reading glasses on so I can't tell. That'd be a shitty life for an exotic sea creature, caught in a tube in a dim windowless room in a crappy industrial estate in Kent.

'Welcome! Lucy, isn't it?'

'Yes, that's me,' I say, trying to be chipper. But since this room has no windows, it feels instantly depressing. It certainly doesn't have a vibe of Vitality, as the workshop is titled. Steve is in his thirties – I'd say thirty-seven, which is too young to be old but too old to be young. He's staring forty in the face and he has an air of desperation about him. He is wearing a crisp white shirt and ironed jeans, with creases so sharp they could chop crudités. I must say, he doesn't look like the cliché I had in mind of a wellness practitioner – dreadlocks and yoga pants – instead he looks like a chirpy estate agent.

'Come in, come in! It's so marvellous to meet you!'

'Thanks!' I say. His tone reminds me of an eighties game show host. I'm trying to match his enthusiasm but it's not easy in this shoebox. 'Erm . . . you too!'

'Leave the door open, can you?'

I'm not surprised he needs the door open. I'm thinking, *Steve: look at your life. You're burning oils in a windowless room, man. Do better.*

I sit down at a round table with him and he starts off by opening up a plastic box with rows of tiny brown-glass bottles, which I assume are the essential oils. I was a teen of the eighties and we were bloody obsessed with essential oils when I was that age. Jacqui and I would go down to the hippy shop in town (where we'd buy hippy skirts and joss sticks) and save up the money we earned at our crappy jobs to buy the latest essential oil and burn it in our increasingly elaborate burners in our bedrooms. My mum always used to enter my room and swipe at the air like she was being attacked by wasps, then stride over to the window and shove it open, come summer or winter.

'Stinks like a house of ill repute in here!' she'd cry and I'd tell her to leave me alone.

So, I know a thing or two about essential oils. Or at least, I used to. Actually, Jacqui and I knew nothing about essential oils and their inherent properties. We just bought the ones that smelt nice or had pretty names. I remember patchouli being a particular favourite, and what was that other one I loved . . . ? Clary sage, that's it. They sounded so romantic. But really they were just a very expensive version of a Glade plug-in.

'Do you vape? You know, vaping?' asks Steve, smiling broadly. He's definitely been abroad for veneers. Nobody has teeth that white. They're so bright, they basically serve as lighting in this miserable coffin of a room.

'I do not, but I've smoked a bit in the past. Gave it up, though. Why would you ask that?'

'Ah ha,' says Steve mysteriously and from a leather wallet, he takes out a bunch of vape pens in a range of neon colours.

'Let me introduce you to my Vitality Vaping and Essential Oils Workshop.'

'Whoa there. Hang on. I wouldn't have come to this if I'd known it was about vaping. I'm massively anti-smoking.'

'Oh, me too,' replies Steve, flashing those veneers again.

'But, the vapes . . . ?' I trail off.

'Oh, these are wellness vapes. No nicotine whatsoever. Nothing harmful in here at all. I can assure you, all you'll be inhaling through these is the goodness of essential elements and minerals your body needs. It's just another interface within the body, like the gut and the skin. We can absorb nutrients through our lungs too. These wellness vapes are the antidote to all smoking and a novel new way to take in important elements that are essential to a healthy body and mind.'

Well, that sounds good. Cigarettes are the devil's work, that's for sure. Maybe wellness vaping might not be as bad as I thought at first.

'I'll begin with a little information about essential oils. Basically, they are ancient miracles. All natural products, put on this planet to heal us and help us. Don't forget, the Three Wise Men brought frankincense and myrrh to our Lord Jesus.'

Oh bloody hell, he's not going to go all Goddy on me, is he? He kept that quiet in the blurb.

'And gold,' I add. 'Arguably more useful, Steve.'

'You're not the first person to make that observation, Lucy!' he quips. 'You might think gold is more precious than these treasures, but you'd be wrong. So wrong, Lucy!'

All right, calm down.

He goes on, 'So tonight I'll be introducing you to a range of wellness vapes, followed by a discussion about essential oils and by the end, I'm sure you'll agree with me about what treasure we have stored in these vital products. We'll begin with our vaping, okay?'

He fans out three coloured vape pens and says, 'The red has the delicious flavour of raspberry, the green matcha and the yellow is mango. But let's find out what goodies lie within these tasty treats.'

'Can I just ask a question, Steve?'

'Of course, Lucy.'

Why do we keep using each other's names all the time? I can't stop doing it! We sound like co-anchors on an American morning show. Steve certainly has the teeth for it.

'Steve, can you explain to me why inhaling anything into your lungs is a good idea? I mean, as far as I know, we get our vitamins and minerals through the gut from food.'

'We do, Lucy. But think about how the lungs take in oxygen for our bodies. So they can take anything else in too, including the goodness of B12 and many other wellness-enhancing elements from vaping.'

'Okay . . .' I reply, doubtfully. I don't know. I'm sure lungs weren't designed to inhale mango-flavoured mist, whatever Steve says.

'So,' Steve unfailingly goes on, 'here we have some of the most health-giving vapes on the market, which I get exclusively from a special supplier in Finland. These are the purest vapes you can buy and each one of them has specific contents that are aimed at a range of bodily processes to give you a pure hit of vitality. The yellow one here is a B12 vape, which targets fatigue and dizziness. The green is melatonin, which ends sleep disturbances and creates a calm and peaceful night's slumber. The red here is milk thistle, known to be effective in reducing the effects of liver ailments, diabetes and cancer. And here we have . . .'

'I'm going to stop you there, Steve, if you don't mind,' I say. 'Cancer? You're saying a vape can cure cancer?'

'Ah no, Lucy, if only that were true. But milk thistle has been proven to reduce its effects.'

'What kind of effects?'

I'm thinking of my dad. And the lung cancer that took him from us, too young, too soon. And now this idea of wellness vaping is making me feel sick.

'An array of effects, Lucy. A veritable array. Milk thistle has been shown to be effective in the fight against cancer, through vigorous anecdotal evidence.'

Ah, there's that phrase again, 'anecdotal evidence'. And what the hell is 'vigorous anecdotal evidence'? Were they doing burpees while they talked about milk thistle helping their cancer? And then that's used as evidence for this crap? I could have an out and out row with Steve. But honestly, I'm only here for credit to get a promotion, I have to keep reminding myself.

I stare at the vapes. They look like the colours reserved for kids' sweeties.

'I'm not sure . . . ' I say.

If I let Steve talk me into this, it'd be the first time I've inhaled something other than air in years. Seven years to be precise. I know that because I gave up my casual smoking habit the day Dad was diagnosed with lung cancer. After we knew he wasn't going to make it, I cursed every single cigarette I ever smoked with him. And I felt guilty, horribly guilty, for years, for the sneaky little fags Dad and I used to share out at the bottom of the garden, away from the judgemental glare of Shirl and Mum. They never smoked, either of them. Dad loved to smoke, revelled in it. I wasn't addicted like he was, but I liked one or two with a drink when I was out. The first fag of the evening, alongside the first sip of an ice-cold gin and tonic, there's nothing quite like that. The way the first inhale takes the smoke so deep into your lungs, it feels like it's tickling your tummy. It's warm and comforting and yet wakes you up, makes you tingle and buzz, especially on an empty stomach. My God, it's an evil and visceral pleasure, smoking. I knew it was then, but still liked to partake of an evening, now and then.

When I'd visit the olds it was a fun thing to do, to escape from the women and stroll down the garden arm in arm, past Dad's vegetable patch chaotic with weeds, down to the lean-to greenhouse at the end, beside the garage where he'd tinker with bits of engines, to escape the house. Dad and I seemed to have a wide variety of ways to escape that house. It was as if the house belonged to Mum and Shirl, while the garden and the garage belonged to me and Dad. There was always that divide: us and them. Why was it like that? Why did it have to be that way? I loved Mum and I loved Shirl. My sister and I often shared the same obsessions throughout our childhoods: Sindy horses, Pierrot duvet covers, Holly Hobbie pencil cases. We'd play for hours and hours making up elaborate romances about the three of them: Holly Hobbie was the love child of Sindy and Pierrot who were madly in love but couldn't be together for . . . reasons (different elaborate reasons each time). And I loved my mum, the special puddings she'd make on Sundays, like upside-down pineapple cake which we always had with a scoop of Neapolitan ice cream. Or a lemon sponge which came out of the oven steaming and had a pool of sticky-sweet lemon syrup pooled underneath it. God, they were so good. She laboured in that kitchen, she really did. She was a good mum, she looked after us well, and did what needed to be done. I don't know . . . but somehow, this split between the four of us started as a crack when we were little and it just grew and grew over time, until it was a chasm, which could never be crossed. And when Dad was gone, I'd lost my half, whereas Shirl still had hers. I was so jealous of her for that, green with envy, that she still had Mum and I didn't have Dad. What a terrible waste of time it was for everyone, that divide between us. And still is.

'Come to any conclusions, Lucy?' says Steve, interrupting my reverie.

'What?' I say, still buried in childhood memories.

'Are you going to take the plunge and try a vape?'

'Oh God, no,' I say without thinking.

He makes a sad face, which makes me grimace involuntarily.

'Sure I can't tempt you, Lucy?'

'I am sure as eggs is eggs, Steve. My dad died of lung cancer. Vaping isn't exactly high on my list of things to try.'

I can tell I've shocked him. And I can tell he'd still quite like to assure me that vaping is safe. But he just says he's sorry to hear that and then rather awkwardly pipes up a cheery, 'Moving on!'

He launches straight into a discussion about essential oils. There's a variety of them in his box, from woody-scented anise – which apparently benefits your respiratory and digestive system, as well as your nervous system and, randomly, your tongue and your gums – to the flowery odour of ylang ylang, which Steve says puts your emotional health in tip top condition.

'So, Steve, if I drink a few drops of ylang ylang, I'll be happy as Larry?'

'Oh no, Lucy, never ingest essential oils. These are strictly for external use only. You can put drops on warm towels.'

Ooh, there's those warm towels again. They do a lot of heavy lifting in the wellness world, it seems.

Steve continues, 'Or you can use them in inhalers, or heat them, or you can roll them on like a deodorant. You can add them to a neutral oil and massage them into your skin too.'

'I get a rash from having a shower if it's a degree too hot, Steve, so I'm not sure that's a good idea for me.'

'Oh, don't worry about that, Lucy. Essential oils are never bad for you, for anyone. There has never been any documented evidence that any essential oil has ever given anyone an adverse skin reaction. So, do massage away with any you choose.'

Something tells me that doesn't sound right. There's always someone who's allergic to something. I have weird skin, or so the doctor once told me. I think I'll be avoiding pouring ylang ylang all over myself later, thanks, Steve, as I don't fancy a Friday night in A&E.

'What's your favourite essential oil then, Steve?'

'Hmm, good question, Lucy. There are so many wonderful ones to choose from. But if I had to choose one . . . I'd say cinnamon. It's absolutely brilliant for your immune system. I'm burning that right now. Plus I've mixed a little hint of an oil that promotes melatonin in your body. So you'll get a fabulous night's sleep tonight, Lucy, just you wait and see. Essential oils can cure insomnia for life-long healthy sleep.'

There we have it again, these sweeping statements about health that don't seem to have any basis in reality. How is inhaling an oil made from cinnamon bark going to help you fight off Covid or flu or the norovirus or whatever? I don't believe a word of it. But Steve seems like a nice guy and honestly I can't be bothered to fight with him about it. He believes in his things, I'll believe in mine. But the oils themselves, they don't look too bad for you, I suppose. They're natural, after all. Steve starts talking about all the good essential oils can do in the world.

'You know, Lucy, essential oils aren't just for private usage. They are actually reducing anxiety for people in hospital who've just had major surgery, or helping severely autistic youngsters to calm themselves and get a good night's sleep.'

'That sounds impressive, Steve.'

And I must admit, all of that does sound benign. But Steve goes on and on about everything these miracle drops are supposed to cure, in his opinion. Or not, as Steve tells me these are facts. Diseases, conditions, aches and pains, woes and miseries, anxiety and depression – you name it, there's an essential oil that'll cure it. Then, I start to wonder, what is this part of the therapy about? He hasn't actually used any of the oils with me. We've not actually done anything with them except talk about them. What's his game? For I'm pretty damn sure by now, Steve has a game.

'Lucy,' he says, in a wheedling kind of way that confirms my suspicions that he's going to ask me a favour.

'You want a review on TrustPilot, Steve?' I ask.

Steve chuckles and says, 'Ah, only if you're feeling generous, Lucy! But it's time for me to be generous to you. Because I have something so exciting to share with you, Lucy. An amazing opportunity for you, Lucy.'

Okay, the first-name usage is getting out of hand now.

'For it's not only me who is allowed to sell these excellent Finnish essential oils into the UK market. I'm sure you'll be just thrilled to discover that you, Lucy – yes, you – could be selling these too as a highly lucrative side hustle to your regular job. And let me tell you, I used to be an IT technician in schools but my essential oils work has become so lucrative in my working life that I left my other job in the dust and now I do this full-time!'

'So, you don't have a background in wellness then, Steve. You were actually a computer nerd, before you used your years of expertise to start selling health products?'

'I did indeed and you'd need no previous experience of the wellness industry either, Lucy. Anyone can get involved. Anyone can become a success with these marvellous products, Lucy. There are colleagues of mine I've seen go from a few pounds a week to six-figure salaries in less than five and a half months.'

'That's weirdly specific, Steve.'

'But happens to be true, Lucy. So, all you'd need to do today, Lucy, is sign up for a month's lot of stock and for a small fee you'd buy that stock, and all you'd need to do is find friends and family to buy from you – which I'm sure you'd find an absolute breeze, Lucy! And after all, these products just sell themselves, they really do. And then you'd be eligible for our Wellness Climbers award programme, where you could earn bonuses from Bronze, to Silver, to Gold and what's more . . . '

And so he goes on, for an eternity, banging on about his pathetic little pyramid scheme that, along with his shiny veneered smile, no doubt catches out some poor naïve housewives desperate for a bit of extra cash to pay off their credit cards while he ropes them into his multi-level marketing nightmare. Oh Steve, what a disappointment you've turned out to be. And I was just starting to think you weren't all that bad after all.

I wait until he's finished his spiel and then I say, 'No thanks, Steve. I won't be partaking. I'd rather smear myself in peanut butter and wander naked through a Canadian forest.'

Steve stares at me, not sure if he's meant to laugh or be offended. But then he can't resist flashing his pearly whites at me again, before asking in a voice he presumes is charming, 'Sure I can't tempt you, Lucy?'

'Oh, do piss off, Steve.'

Even after that, he shakes my hand enthusiastically and bids me a good night. I drive away from the sad little industrial estate, stinking of an unholy melange of odours.

When I get home, I message Jacqui to see if she's up for a phone call debrief and she replies that she will be in twenty minutes or so.

While I'm waiting, I sit on the sofa, the telly on for comfort in the background. I google some stuff about essential oils and find out Steve was right about hospitals, as some do use them to help with anxiety. But I also search up the dangers of skin reactions and find plenty of evidence that some people have had really nasty rashes from essential oils. Oh, Steve, you shitty little liar, you. But I can't say I didn't enjoy our session tonight. I enjoyed hearing about the essential oils, though what actual benefits they have, I'm still at a bit of a loss. And whatever the health advantages might be of wellness vaping – and I'm not convinced of a single jot of it – it did give me a chance to have a think about stuff. I read more stuff about essential oils and all the people that swear by them. Plus how many pyramid schemes they've unfortunately spawned.

Then Jacqui calls.

'Hit me,' she says.

'Sure you've got enough time?'

'Yeah, the kids are murdering each other on the Xbox and I've got a glass of red, so happy days. What was Steve the oilman like?'

I tell her the ins and outs of Steve's pitch.

'It wasn't the worst hour I've ever spent in my life, I suppose,' I conclude. 'But I can't believe I spent £150 on that! One hundred and fifty English pounds!'

'Well, I'm not surprised,' says Jacqui. 'That's cheap for this wellness stuff.'

'How do you know?'

'I do actually know things, you know! I am a journalist! I've covered wellness a couple of times for the paper. I did some stuff on a new wellness centre in Sittingbourne last year. Plus I covered a court case about a wellness scammer.'

'What's a wellness scammer?'

'Oh Christ, the whole industry is rife with it. Some of the worst scammers out there are wellness scammers. Basically, it's like the modern version of snake oil and these scammers don't pull any punches. They're clever, and manipulative, and they work on your fears and your needs and desperation. They'll lie and lie and lie to get what they want. Some of them are multi-millionaires. Some of them are in prison. I know we're laughing now, but keep your wits about you, Lu. These wellness scammers are the *worst*.'

I've never heard of this. I mean, I know there are scammers everywhere, but I didn't realise how widespread it was in this field.

'But surely they're not all scammers or grifters, are they? I think I just assumed that they actually believe in this woo-woo stuff themselves.'

'Some of them do,' says Jacqui. 'Okay, so, you know when I had that back pain and it went down my arm and I was in agony? And I had that electroacupuncture? It was the only thing that worked, remember. Changed my life.'

I remember it, how bad she was back then. She could barely move.

'But that's not scammy wellness stuff, is it?' I ask. 'I think of acupuncture like ancient wisdom. I think even GPs recommend it now, don't they?'

'Well, some might. But you could still say it's part of the wellness industry spectrum, I suppose. And my mum, one of her best friends is a Reiki healer and she goes to see her regularly.'

'I've heard of that. But that's just massage, isn't it?'

'Not really. The hands are held above the body. It's about manipulating energy. Now, some sceptics might call that a load of old shite. But my mum's friend believes in it, and so does Mum. And she's always one hundred per cent better afterwards in herself, physically and mentally. It really works for her. It actually makes her less aggravating for a while, so it's got my thumbs up too.'

'I ought to recommend it to Shirley. Well, either stuff like Reiki is real – and who are we to know either way? There's more in heaven and earth than your philosophy, Horatio, and all that. Or it's the placebo effect. I suppose it doesn't really matter, if it works.'

'Exactly. And that's what the wellness industry is based on. And a lot of the scammier stuff doesn't work at all, or could even be harmful. So, I'd say, keep an open mind to some of it, as hilarious as this lot sounds. And this Rejuvenate course thing sounds fucking nuts! So it's also really important to keep a healthy scepticism before you part with a lot of money.'

After our call, later in bed, I'm lying awake thinking about this wellness stuff – is it all a scam? Or is there something to it? Could we be living happier, healthier lives just by buying a few products off a bloke in an industrial estate? Once I've gnawed on that bone for a while, I think about work and how it would feel to get my dream promotion and how proud Dad would've been if he could see me reach the pinnacle of my career. He'd have been proud as punch. If it happens, Mum and Shirl's reactions would probably be a shrug. Then I can't stop thinking about Dad and me, and Mum and Shirl. And I'm awake and tossing and turning half the night about that one. I don't get to sleep till gone 3am. So, the melatonin oil didn't work too well on sleeplessness, did it, Steve?

Chapter 7

'Your name is actually Yorick? That's on your birth certificate?'

Surely – SURELY – he just nicked that name from doing *Hamlet* at school.

'That's right,' says Yorick and smiles. There's a certain kind of wellness smile. It's friendly, insincere and smug all at once.

Here I am in my third wellness session in three weeks. I actually found I was looking forward to this one, not because I thought it'd do me any good – it has the ridiculous title of Fossil Therapy, for fuck's sake – but because it does at least get me out of the house and away from work. I don't do enough of that, if I'm honest with myself. So, here I am, on a Thursday night at seven, in a therapy room in the arts centre in Tonbridge. There's a candle burning that smells like Vosene shampoo. The furniture is minimal and in the centre of the room is a chair that looks like something from a dentist's garage sale. Other than that, the room is plain and lacking in character – unlike Yorick, who has long curly hair pulled into a rough ponytail, and a significant beard, and is wearing the classic wellness garb of patchwork trousers, a baggy linen shirt and a leather waistcoat. I'm still having fun with his name. With Boudicca, all this wellness stuff was new to me and I was rather polite. Now I've been doing this for three weeks, I'm starting to find my feet and I can't resist ribbing this walking cliché about his daft name.

'Like Hamlet holding the skull: *Alas, poor Yorick. I knew him well*,' I say in a mock dramatic voice.

'*Alas, poor Yorick, I knew him, Horatio*, actually. Most people misquote that line,' Yorick replies and there's that smile again.

'Touché, Yorick. Were your parents big Shakespeare fans then?'

'They were both actors and loved the theatre. My sister is called Mousetrap.'

'Really?!'

Yorick laughs. 'No. I'm just kidding.'

We both laugh. 'You got me there, Yorick!'

'Good,' he says and chuckles good-naturedly. Then I realise I've actually been quite rude.

'I apologise, Yorick, for commenting on your name. I'm a director of HR and I should know better. I'm sorry.'

'Hey, that's all right. I often get comments on it. I was bullied mercilessly at school. I'm used to it!'

'That's no excuse for me though,' I say and genuinely mean it.

Of the two of us, I'm the one who's been a bit of an arsehole tonight so far. Despite his appearance, Yorick actually seems like the most down-to-earth of the three wellness types I've met so far. My usual age-pinpointing talent is challenged tonight. His clothes look like he was a child of the seventies, like me. But his lack of wrinkles and grey hair suggest he's probably in his late twenties, early thirties. I wonder what his parents think of his job? Maybe they're old hippies, who did Woodstock and brought Yorick up in a travelling theatre troupe, who knows. Either way, he's making a small fortune out of this fossil stuff and could very well keep them in their old age, charging £150 an hour to do something weird with fossils.

'Shall we begin?' says Yorick.

'Yes, let's.'

Yorick leads me over to the deep window sill where, displayed in a long row, is a wide variety of fossils. They really are rather lovely. I've liked fossils for a long time, since family holidays to Dorset, the bit they now call the Jurassic Coast. There are beaches like Charmouth and Burton Bradstock where you can simply pick up fossils from the beach, lying all around you, everywhere. I used to bring them home and Dad would varnish them to make them shine. I've still got a couple in a bowl of shells in my house. Reminds me of happier times. Yorick's collection is far more impressive: not simply the odd ammonite and trilobite, spiral-shaped and flat shells, plus much rarer specimens, such as tiny fish and prehistoric plants perfectly preserved in astonishing detail.

'May I touch them?'

'Of course.'

I pick up an ammonite and hold it in the centre of my palm. I wonder how many millions of years ago this creature once flitted about the oceans.

'I've always loved fossils, Yorick. They give me the history shivers.'

'Yup,' says Yorick. 'They're like time machines. Wonderful

things. As some of the oldest critters on our beautiful planet, their ancient wisdom can now guide us.'

Ah, here comes the wellness spiel in all its scammy glory. Shame, as we were getting on famously.

Yorick continues, 'Holding fossils close to ourselves can give us insights about our bodies and our minds. Their ancient wisdom enables us to read our internal organs and draw conclusions about how to improve our health.'

'You can tell all that from a fossil?'

'Absolutely. They have miraculous qualities. The therapy I've developed with fossils is designed to reset your "brain-flux", which is our brain's ability to communicate effectively with the rest of our bodies. Our brain-flux isn't working to its optimal levels. Nobody's is. In this modern world, we spend far too much time obsessing over things that don't matter, while ignoring our deeper knowledge. Our brain-flux is out of whack. Our modern brains are not sending the right codes to our body parts. After this session, you should feel over a hundred per cent better optimised. Would you like to take a seat?'

I move over to the repurposed dentist's chair in the centre of the room and wonder what on earth he's going to do with those fossils. Fossils are great. But his spiel reached new depths of bullshit wellness double-speak. Everything is vague, nothing is provable and it all sounds the same as every other spiel. They're magical, they're a cure-all, they're ancient wisdom. And after such a promising opening of witty wordplay, I'm now rather disappointed with Yorick. Urgh, okay, let's get this over with.

I sit down on the dentist's chair, which is rather comfy. After that, it just gets weirder. Yorick turns down the dimmer switch so that the room isn't so bright. He puts on some light classical music, then explains what's going to happen next.

'I'll be selecting a range of different fossils and holding them in the air above your person. Each fossil is directed at a different zone of your body. When it comes in contact with your aura, the fossil will draw negative rays from your past traumas and maladapted internal organs out of your body and direct them into the fossil. There the fossil will catch and keep those negative vibrations, absorb them, then throw each one back into history, where it will dissipate in the winds of time.'

I don't . . . I don't even know what to say to that avalanche of verbal diarrhoea. Still, Yorick seems so earnest, I feel churlish.

'Are we ready?' he says.

I nod. Here we go.

Yorick picks up different fossils and waves each one slowly over various parts of my body. He starts with my nose, then my ears and eyes. He then waves a few more fossils, his hand hovering over each of my vital organs for a while. A couple of times during this charade, he makes little noises in his throat, as if there's a kind of wind resistance against his hand and he has to edge the fossil forward in the air to enable it to do its job, especially over my ribs area. Wow, he's really committed to making this look legit. At one point, he seems to really struggle with one fossil, hovering over my upper right abdomen.

'Everything all right, Yorick?'

'Sure, don't worry. I'll get there.'

He makes another noise of struggle and then eases the fossil through the air and further down my body, smiling and nodding as he does so.

'What was the issue there then?'

'You have a hell of a lot of resistance in your body, Lucy. Especially in your liver. Your lungs were pretty clogged up too. But don't worry, I dissipated the negative energy in both. You should feel much freer in those regions after the therapy.'

He carries on, doing both legs and my feet. I'm thinking about what he said, about my liver and my lungs. It gives me a shiver up my spine. How did he know that just a few months ago, my GP told me my liver function blood test results weren't great? And what Yorick said about my lungs. Could he have known that my lungs are a source of anxiety for me, due to the disease that killed my dad? It's weird, yes, this whole business of Yorick's Fossil Therapy, but also rather pleasant. The room is dim, the music is nice and it's actually so relaxing having someone waving their arms gently and lovingly over your body. I decide to go with it and close my eyes. Gosh, it just feels so nice lying here. I have no responsibilities at this moment, no demands on my attention. Yorick is doing his stuff and I'm just here vibing. I'm glad this isn't like a normal massage. I had one of those once and found it a deeply uncomfortable experience. Not just the physical aspect of it hurting quite a bit, especially around my shoulders, but the actual fact of a complete stranger laying hands all over me . . . I know it's normal and people have massages all the time, but I pretty much hated it. Never again. This is different though. No touching here. And no hassle. Just fossils and vibrations and a chilled-out mood.

When we're done, I'm quite disappointed. Yorick turns up the dimmer switch and floods the room with light, which feels unwelcome. I'd much rather stay in the dimness.

'How was that?' says Yorick, smiling.

'You know what, I really enjoyed that!'

And I actually mean it! I did!

'Good, good. We did some useful work here today. There was a deep backlog of opposition between your body and your mind, so the brain-flux had to work really hard to do its job. I think you'll find your thoughts come easier tonight. You should feel much freer, more relaxed, as your brain-flux is relaxed now. Like a blockage in a pipe. It's dissipated now and will flow freely.'

It all sounds so nice. I wish I could believe him.

'Where did this fossil idea come from? Is it yours?' I ask him.

'Yeah,' he says, taking hold of his long ponytail and tugging on it thoughtfully. 'I've known since I was a child that I had a profound connection to ancient places. When I held my first fossil, it just buzzed through me like it was alive. I dropped it! I was scared shitless! Then, when I was a bit older, I got into Reiki healing. And I realised I could marry the two things and hopefully, really help people.'

'Ah, I've heard of Reiki. My friend's mum goes to Reiki regularly and loves it apparently.'

'I used to practise Reiki too, but that's about channelling energy into your body, not drawing it out. Either way, both Fossil Therapy and Reiki are really about love. The fossils love us, energy loves us, the Great Creator loves us. They're all about love.'

It all sounds so nice. But also flaky and daft. I've often wondered how nice it would be to believe in God, but I never managed it. Atheist through and through. Now I'm wondering about some of this more far out wellness stuff, like Yorick's schtick. But, to be fair, he seems so genuine.

'Yorick, do you mind me asking something about you?'

'Sure, I don't mind,' he says. He's not particularly charming, Yorick. He's just quite matter of fact, not trying to persuade you of anything. Or alternatively that's the schtick he's developed to make himself seem more legit. It's impossible to tell.

'Do you believe in this stuff? I mean, really? Look I'm never coming back here – I'm only doing it to get a promotion at work. If you tell me, I won't tell a soul.'

He laughs at that. 'So you think my therapy will manifest this new job?'

'Oh blimey, no. I was just competing with this rival woman at work and she was doing this wellness month thing, so I lied and said I was doing it too to impress my bosses.'

'Ah, I see. Subterfuge and deceit. That won't get you anywhere in life, Lucy.'

He's smiling, not looking judgy. But I do feel a little bit of judgement.

'Well, we shall see about that, won't we, Yorick! Maybe I'll come back when I've got the job and book ten sessions! I could afford it then!'

We both laugh. Then I remember, he still hasn't answered my question. 'You believe in it then, all this fossil stuff?'

'I absolutely believe it.'

And I believe him. I mean, I believe that he believes it. I don't. There's no way a bunch of bits of old rock could have any effect on your body or mind or anything at all.

'Thanks, Yorick, for being such a good sport.'

'Thank you, Lucy, for keeping an open mind. Oh, and I have one more thing to show you, before we're done.'

He picks up a small rucksack from a chair and places it

on a table, pulling from it a slim box filled with some sort of packaged snacks.

'It's a wellness energy bar I've designed myself, made from health-giving ingredients such as dried Tibetan goji berries, high-cocoa-percentage dark chocolate, gluten-free oats, organic walnut butter and omega 3-infused chia seeds, along with a range of customised supplements of key vitamins and minerals that I've chosen for you based on your brain-flex reading today. It'll settle the effects of the therapy in your body and ensure its effects are optimised.'

He hands the energy bar to me. It has the exact same spiel written on it that Yorick has just rattled off to me. He must've learnt it by heart.

'How can it be customised to me,' I ask, 'if you've just pulled it from your bag randomly, Yorick, eh?'

'Not randomly. I've developed a range of these supplement bars in different categories. Yours is related to liver and lung health, see? It says it here on the side.'

It does, I can see that. But, of course, he could've said liver and lungs during the reading to match the energy bar. And then it hits me: before the session, I had to fill in a questionnaire and there were pretty detailed questions on there, particularly about how much alcohol you drink and how much you smoke, or used to. Plus medical conditions that run in the family. So that's how he knew it was pretty likely I might have issues with my liver and my lungs. Sneaky devil.

'Thanks, Yorick,' I say, with a sigh. I have no intention of eating this rubbish, but I go to pop it in my handbag to be polite.

'Ah no, sorry, that's to purchase as an extra, if you wish. That'll be £15 please.'

'Fifteen quid for a snack?!' I cry.

'It's a customised energy bar and I assure you, it'll be worth the money.'

I've given Yorick the benefit of the doubt so far but now I'm just annoyed.

'Yorick, you really have disappointed me with this, you know. I enjoyed the session and now you're giving me the hard sell on this nonsense? I've already paid you plenty of money!'

Yorick shrugs his shoulders and smiles. He says, good-naturedly, 'This is my business. I have to make a living. Plus I know this energy bar will help you embed the hard work we've done here today.'

'You actually believe in these supplement bars too?'

'I do. I eat them myself, every day without fail.'

'No wonder you need to grift then. They cost a fortune!'

Yorick laughs and replies, 'Well, I get them at wholesale price, but that's not the point. They really do work. Conventional medicine is not the only way and it often lets us down. We must reclaim our heirloom knowledge of natural medicine. It helped us survive as a species for thousands of years. Western medicine is relatively young in comparison and yet we set it up like a god. Think about it, Lucy. Who would you rather trust for their wisdom, a child or an old woman?'

The next person knocks on the door and I have to go. I firmly place the overpriced energy bar back on the table, then take my leave. As I'm going out of the door, Yorick calls out, 'Don't forget to follow me on Instagram, Lucy!'

Despite his hard sell moment at the end, Yorick has really made me think, especially with that last comment. After all, we do believe a lot of the time that modern medicine will cure us and yet, so often, it fails us. Drugs don't work for some people, or they have horrible side effects, or some medical professionals gaslight us or ignore us or patronise us. Why do we put so much faith in modern medicine, when it is such a recent phenomenon? Maybe we're still like our distant ancestors, early humans, throwing rocks at the sun, and blindly following our religion we've created, peopled with its priests as GPs, nurses, consultants and surgeons? I never thought in a million years that some guy in patchwork trousers waving fossils at me would make me question something I'd taken for granted all of my life. And more to the point, something that I relied on and thought would save my dad.

But it didn't.

Chapter 8

The next day is the last day of the working week, thank God, as I'm so ready for the weekend. I'm seeing Jacqui tomorrow for lunch and can't wait. The morning drags by with a disciplinary meeting for bolshy Barry from Sales who has been reported by his team for sharing YouTube videos in support of Greg Wallace and Russell Brand on the team WhatsApp account, which was bad enough, but then he messaged the woman in his team who reported him that she was a 'dreadful old nag with more wrinkles than a bollock-bag'. So yes, I suspect Barry won't be with us much longer. A blessing for all, but not easy to sit there and listen to him ranting on about the undermining of middle-class men in the workplace and how he feels victimised. I mean, where do you start with these cretins? It's simply not fair that I have to be professional in the face of such poisonous guff. What I really want to do is punch his lights out.

Anyway, after escaping from that, I'm meeting with Nick Bridges this afternoon, which I'm looking forward to, as

I have the chance to really impress him with my wellness stuff, plus all the other work I've been doing at Beane & Co over the last few years. I'm so glad of the opportunity to have a one-to-one. I get into the conference room early, so I can arrange all my paperwork in neat piles for him to look at, plus I've got a PowerPoint to show him on ideas for workplace health initiatives, something I started last year but now I've added wellness buzzwords I've gleaned from my three sessions so far. I'm particularly glad Tara won't be there to interrupt. I'm setting up my PowerPoint when the door opens and I think, Nick's early, but then I look up and it isn't Nick, it's Tara bloody Harryman.

'Tara?' I say, politely as I can, but annoyed, as she shouldn't be here and I don't want her here.

'Lucy, I've been meaning to catch you. How's the January Rejuvenate going for you so far?'

It's three overpriced charlatans touting a great, steaming pile of shite, actually, Tara. That's what I want to say.

'Really super, thanks, Tara. I had Fossil Therapy last night with Yorick. Have you signed up for that one?'

She shakes her head and her pristine red bob doesn't move an inch, welded into place with hairspray.

'No, I didn't pick that one,' she says and there's that smug look again. It seems to keep happening: the ones I've chosen are the ones she hasn't and that look makes me feel that I've made dumb choices. The only one we've had in common is Clarity with Clio, but I can't talk about that yet as I haven't been. Then Tara adds, 'How was it?'

But suddenly, I'm tired of all this bullshit, trying to impress Tara. What do I care what she thinks of me anyway? She's not the one making the decision about my promotion. I'm sick of saying all the right things. The important thing is to impress Nick Bridges and keep Derek on side.

'I thought it was a load of bollocks.'

I watch her reaction carefully. She doesn't react but I'm convinced she's holding back a smile. Suddenly, I have the urge to challenge this pretence between us and dig deeper.

I add, 'What do you think of all this wellness stuff? Do you *really* believe in it, Tara?'

'Not all of it,' Tara says. 'Just like anything in life, the wellness industry has its charlatans.'

That's exactly the word I was thinking of. Now, this is getting interesting.

'I absolutely agree. But doesn't the wellness industry seem to have more charlatans than most?'

'I wouldn't say so, no. I believe most people in life are just trying to do their best for others.'

Could she really be that naïve? Surely she knows most people are rotten. Just look at Barry from Sales, for example. I have to deal with wankers like that every day.

'I think the opposite,' I reply. 'I think that most people in life are shitty. Just look at the comments section of any average public Facebook post. I want most people to just leave me alone.'

Tara gives me that smug smile again, which drives me up the wall. Then she says something that blows me away. 'Maybe that's why you're lonely.'

What? What?! Did she . . . actually say that?

'Lonely? I'm . . . I am not lonely!' I cry, incensed. 'Who says I'm lonely?'

'Everyone,' says Tara, blithely. She folds her arms and looks me right in the eye. 'You're famous for it in the office.

Maybe your loneliness would subside if you let more people in. I think you might actually gain something from January Rejuvenate. At least it gets you away from work and home. It might do you some good, even though you're only doing it to compete with me.'

How fucking dare she! I'm raging. Even though, technically, she's one hundred per cent right about it all. But how does she know? What have people been saying about me? Do they all think I'm some kind of loser? That enrages me even more.

'That's a highly unprofessional thing to say, Tara. It's the kind of thing I might well report to the CEO.'

'You won't do that,' she says with confidence. 'Because it'll make you look petty. And it'll play into the bitch-fight narrative that Derek wants to see. And neither of us wants that, do we?'

Fucking hell, she's right about that. But she's not right about everything.

'You may have a point there but you are still completely out of order, Tara. Firstly, it's nobody's business but mine what I do outside work. And secondly, you don't know me and neither does anyone here at work. I keep myself to myself. And I work bloody hard. And all right, I did do this wellness bullshit to keep up with you. This COO post has been my dream job for years. And I'm damned if I'm going to let you waltz in here and take it from me.'

Tara is cool as a cucumber. She doesn't snap back at me. She just smiles that infuriating little smile of hers again.

'Good,' she says. 'Much better to get these things out in the open. Now we both know where we are with each other, we can get on with it like professionals. May the best woman win.'

I try to think of a witty retort but she's already walked away. Then, Nick Bridges hails Tara in the corridor and they talk and laugh and laugh and talk for about ten minutes, while I'm waiting for him in the conference room, absolutely seething, and sweating, and feeling a bit dizzy and shaky from the shock of what just occurred. Once I've managed to calm down a little bit, I can see what's happening here. She's trying to psych me out. Well, it won't bloody work, Tara. I am up for this fight and I'm going to win, even if I die trying, for fuck's sake. In comes Nick and I plaster on my best management smile and impress the hell out of him with my PowerPoint and my paperwork and my ideas and strategies for an hour straight. Beat that, Tara.

That night I collapse in bed at nine and fall straight to sleep. That's not like me. But this week has shattered me, in more ways than one. Normally, I'd message Jacqui straight away after a work showdown like that one I had with Tara. But I'm too tired for all the back-and-forth messaging, so I decide to keep it for when I see Jacqui tomorrow for lunch.

The next day is Saturday and I have a luxurious morning in bed with the weekend papers, some croissants and jam and the TV news on in the background – my Saturday routine, which I love after a hard week's graft. But actually, I find myself ignoring all of my usual weekend comforts and instead I'm looking at Instagram. First, I scan through Tara's posts. I never post on Instagram. I'm only on it for the memes but otherwise I loathe it and all its narcissistic wank. Her posts are again identical to her other socials. All wellness focused and business queen and all that shite. Makes me sick. Then I find Yorick on Instagram. His feed is full of reels of him explaining how toxic the modern world is and touting his workshops and his madly overpriced energy supplement bars. I then do a search under the term 'wellness' and try to draw some conclusions about what comes up. What I find is a huge variety of stuff, but with some common themes. It's overwhelmingly being touted by women, for women. There's loads of stuff on menopause supplements, the latest wonder-drug of pills or potions to solve all your menopausal woes in one handy capsule or vial or teaspoon. There are pictures of women's bodies in bikinis before and after whatever wellness course they're selling and the women are always standing in weirdly uncomfortable poses that make them look like they need a shit and have to hold it in before getting to the loo on time. There are women at the gym looking at you over their shoulder, while their arses are so unnaturally big they take up the rest of the frame. The word *secrets* comes up a hell of a lot. I mean, it's everywhere. *Top ten wellness secrets*; *three health secrets your doctor doesn't want you to know about*; *I got hotter when I turned fifty due to this one wellness secret*, etc. etc. It all smacks of hidden knowledge that will be revealed to you if you just like and follow. Other key words are *toxic*, *detox*, *alternative*, *integrative*, *holistic*, *life-changing*, *micro-habits*, *hacking your health*, *sleep hygiene*, and *brain resets*. And every image I click reveals a handsome guy or pretty woman selling me something at the kind of exorbitant prices that would make an oligarch think twice.

It's bewildering, all these different methods and approaches and secrets and hacks and after a while I realise I'm having a really grim reaction to it. After doom-scrolling wellness Instagram accounts, my overwhelming feeling is that . . . I feel like shit. I feel like the world's biggest loser. I feel unhealthy, idle and worthless. I feel like my life is on the wrong track, that everything I do is contributing towards my early death, and that I'm the only one who can change my life and yet I'm too stuck in bad old habits that make me sicker and sicker. I look down at my tired old body and I have to agree. What the hell am I doing with my life? I get out of bed and look at the flaky pastry remains of my croissant breakfast on the tray on the bed, the knife smeared with jam, the plate glistening with grease . . . and I feel sick with myself. I'm a bad person. I am morally corrupt. I have let myself become a mess through ignoring the wisdom of the ancients and not only that, the secrets of the Instagram wellness influencers who will put me firmly on the right track to optimising my life – mind, body and soul.

Hang on . . . what the actual FUCK am I talking about?! My God, see how easy it is to get sucked into this stuff? *They* make you feel like shit. *They* make you feel they have the answers to stop you feeling like shit. Only by listening to them – and more importantly, paying them – will you find your way to your highest level of wellbeing. Without it, you're just a useless piece of shit. Blimey, this wellness culture stuff is powerful. But then the doubts come in . . . maybe there's truth in it. Maybe I am screwing up my life, with my takeaways and red wine and chocolate, with my workaholic lifestyle and lack of brisk walks or gym membership. Despite the influencer bullshit, maybe underneath I will be a better person if I seek a new way of living. Or is it all a grift to part me from my money to fill their activewear pockets?

I know what I need. I need a chat with Jacqui. She'll set me straight. She always does. Thank heavens we have our lunch date planned for later today. We're meeting up at our favourite café in Tunbridge Wells that does the best tuna and cheese ciabatta melts in town.

I get there a bit early and have a look at the menu, trying to decide if I should have my usual caramel latte or their seasonal winter warmer of peppermint white chocolate mocha . . . hmmm . . . but then, the imagery of all those skinny women with perfect abs and huge buttocks swim before my eyes. They're not eating paninis and drinking mochas, are they, eh? They're having chia seeds and avocado and protein shakes and green tea. Oh God, I feel miserable again. I can't even enjoy my usual lunch with Jacqui. What's happening to me? I fucking hate this. I'm realising that all this wellness stuff, which just started as a kind of dare, to beat my work rival and get my dream promotion, is starting to take a hold over me. I've seen a gazillion images like these ones before, as they're all over the media and have been forever, even back in the seventies when I grew up, they were in magazines and TV ads and billboards. But somehow now it's worse with social media in our hands and head twenty-four-seven and though I've ignored it in the past, it's now infected my brain and I cannot see past it. I feel utterly suffused with worthlessness and guilt. Then, I think of Tara and her wellness warrior bullshit and I'm suddenly so envious of her, I can't see straight. A terrible fear grips me that she's already got the promotion, that she's a shoo-in and I'm putting myself through all this wellness nonsense for nothing. But worse than that, I deserve to not get that promotion, as Tara is morally and physically superior to me in every way. Because I am a pointless lump of nothingness.

'Cheer up, love, it might never happen!' I hear behind me

and turn to see my lovely friend. I get up quickly from my window seat at the café and give her a big hug and I hang on far longer than normal.

Jacqui knows me too well and whispers, 'Hey . . . what's up, lovely?'

I find when I pull back, I have tears in my eyes. 'Oh Jac, I'm so glad you're here.'

Jacqui sits me down and takes my hand.

'What is it, Lu? Is it about your dad? Missing him?'

Only Jacqui understands how much I still think about my dad, day in, day out, despite it being seven years now. Time doesn't seem to matter when it comes to my grief. It just means I miss him more, as my memory fades and I feel he's further away from me than ever.

'Not today, no. Something else. I just . . . I don't know how to explain it. I just feel . . . crap. About myself.'

Jacqui looks perplexed and squeezes my hand. 'What's happened? This isn't like you. You're so kickass, my darling. You always have been. What's going on? Is it about work?'

Then, I sob. A teenage couple drinking their hot chocolates piled with marshmallows stare at me and snigger.

'What are you laughing at?' Jacqui barks at them. And I love her for that. But I don't want to be in this café anymore.

'Can we go somewhere else?' I say quietly.

'Sure,' she says and holds my hand tightly as we get the hell out of there. Outside on the pavement, she asks me, 'Where do you want to go, love? There's that nice pizza place down there you like. How about there?'

'Oh God, no, not pizza,' I say. I can't bear the thought of food, or at least, unhealthy food. 'Can we just walk a bit?'

'Course. Let's head over to Calverley Grounds. It's only ten minutes from here and we can have a little stroll around the park. We're both wrapped up warm. It'll be nice.'

So, that's what we do. And on the way, I tell her all about Tara's attack. I call it that, because honestly, that's how it felt. I'm used to antagonism at work but I've never felt any adversary at work was worthy of the fight, until now. Tara has really put the wind up me.

'Well, of course you're upset about what that mega bitch said to you!' says Jacqui. 'We all know there are people at work who we hate. And that we have rivals. But you don't say it out loud! We keep it buried inside and let it fester there and poison our souls, like every other healthy British person does!'

That makes me laugh-cry – good old Jacqui. But there's more to tell. I explain how I don't know where these crappy feelings have come from, all of a sudden. How I'm generally happy with my life and with myself. Yes, I want that promotion pretty desperately, but other than that, I'm just not a depressive type of person and generally I enjoy myself, most of the time. And the thought that everyone at work thinks I'm a lonely old hag has really upset me. Then, I tell her about how jealous I am of Tara and how rubbish the wellness stuff on Instagram made me feel and then I say, 'And even that nonsense the other night with that Yorick fossil person . . . ' I burst into tears.

She puts her arm around me and we keep walking, at my insistence, because I know if I stop walking now, I'll weep properly, like I'll totally blub and wail in the street and I don't want that. If I keep putting one foot in front of the other, it takes my mind off wanting to cry like a newborn. We enter the park through the main entrance off Mount Pleasant

Avenue. It feels really good to be walking in the chill air. The trees are bare of leaves and their jagged limbs stand starkly against the blue sky, while the winter sun thinly shines on the ornamental beds and landscaping of the park. Jacqui and I both have scarves and gloves on, with a raspberry beret for Jacqui (yes, from the song and yes, she even bought it from a second-hand store, which made us laugh when she found it and we sang the Prince song so loudly we were told we were bothering the other customers) and I'm wearing a bobble hat which I now feel ridiculous in. Maybe I'm too old for a bobble hat. Urgh, I don't know anymore. I feel like all my clothes are stupid and make me look stupid, all of a sudden.

'What happened with this Yorick person then?' asks Jacqui. 'Was he mean to you? Did he do anything . . . you know . . . weird?'

'Oh God, no. I mean, yeah, the fossil waving was by its very nature weird. But he wasn't *weird* weird. He was fine. I enjoyed it actually. It was just what he said after this ridiculous fossil body scan thing. I know it's a load of rubbish. But he said that there was something wrong with my liver and my lungs. And that frightened me. And even though I knew that he'd just used the information from my questionnaire to make it seem like he had found out these secrets of my body, it really made me worry. About what I'm doing to my body. About my dad's body. And maybe history repeating itself. I don't know. It's just really upset me. And then when I looked at all that wellness stuff this morning . . . and it hit me, that maybe I am a wreck. And need to change my life or something. But how can I do it quickly enough to beat Tara? Perfect bloody Tara with the perfect bloody life? I don't know . . . it just got to me. And I feel rotten. I'm sorry.'

'What are you sorry about?!' cries Jacqui and puts both arms around my shoulders and squeezes really hard. 'You've got nothing to be sorry for. You've had a bit of a shock and it made you think of your dad. No wonder you're upset.'

'Maybe that's all it is then,' I say pensively, as we walk slowly down the path. Despite the cold January air, it's so calming to be out here, amongst the grass and trees. There's a bed of hellebores over there, they're my favourite. They always make me think of new life coming in spring. Mum planted some in the front garden at our old house. She liked them too. I don't suppose they have hellebores in New Zealand, or do they? Maybe I'll ask her. I'm really glad Jacqui and I left that café and came out here. It's a real tonic. Trees, sky, the chill air.

'Well, you say that like it's nothing,' says Jacqui, dragging me back to reality. 'And it's not nothing. You're still dealing with missing your dad. And the complicated stuff with your family. And yes, even Martin leaving. I know it's years ago but that doesn't mean you're not still dealing with it. Plus now, the job stuff is bringing it all into focus, I think. Work has been the one constant in all that huge change you've had to deal with. You've always been able to rely on it. And now this bloody Tara Whats-her-face has glided in on her killer heels and threatened everything you've been working towards for years. No wonder you're feeling like crap.'

'Well yes, once you put it like that,' I reply. 'Fuck a duck, you're a good therapist, Jac. Have you ever thought about shifting career?!'

'Ha ha! Well, I have to be as a mum, especially to teens. They need constant therapy. And I need constant therapy to deal with them and their constant, all-consuming dramas, the little fuckers.'

We laugh at that. Jacqui really does wring herself dry for those kids. Barna is great too and is a good dad and husband. But Jacqui is the one they always turn to when they're suffering. They're so lucky to have her. So lovely to have a mum with empathy. And I know that well, because my mum never had much.

'But listen,' says Jacqui, linking arms and pulling me close. 'You are going to get through this. I'm still certain you'll get this job. You have all the qualifications and experience necessary and nobody knows that place as well as you do. And the last thing you need, while you're under the strain of preparing for the conference and impressing the new boss, is scrolling through Instagram and comparing yourself to all the gym bunnies on there with their fake filters and perfect lighting and AI to give them unearthly beauty. You know it's all fake on there, don't you? Everybody knows it. But it's like your brain and your eyes don't confer and you end up feeling like crap when you're looking at these aliens. Because they are aliens. They're not human. They're not real. And the lifestyles they brag about aren't real either. Nobody really lives that way, they're not really eating perfect food and doing perfect workouts all the time. What you don't see is when they're stress-eating a KitKat, all four fingers in their gob at once. They don't put that on Instagram! Honey, *everyone* feels shit when they doom-scroll on Instagram.'

I'm laughing now and holding on to Jacqui for dear life.

'Thank fuck for you, Jac.'

'And thank fuck for you! If I couldn't rant at you about my kids and work and life in general, I'd lose my bloody mind.'

'I worry I don't listen enough! I always feel like you're always listening to my woes and I don't do enough for you.'

'Only because sometimes I just don't want to hear myself drone on about it. That's not your fault. And I'm very protective of you, chick. Ever since your dad . . . and Martin . . . I've got Barna and the kids, after all. It's my job to look out for you.'

'And mine for you. I hope I do enough for you, Jac.'

'Course you do. Look, we middle-class women of a certain age need to stick together, darling. Nobody else is going to fight our battles for us. Society at large thinks we're a waste of space. Too old to fuck, too young to play the wise old crone. We're a joke to most. We have to stand tall and give each other the strength we need. So we can get on with kicking ass. And you will kick ass, Lu. You always do.'

Thank fuck for Jac. Thank fuck for my best friend. For reminding me who I am.

Chapter 9

Thank God this Friday is the last wellness session. Finally, I can gather my notes and start writing up this new wellness nonsense for work, plan the conference speech and nail this job. My last wellness thing is called Clarity with Clio. Yes, Clio with an 'i'. Isn't that the Renault car? 'Nicole? Papa!' and all that? I want to see a birth certificate again! After another long week of hassle, I drive out to a place just outside Langton Green, a nice little village just beyond Rusthall. I'm glad it'll be a quick drive home, as I really cannot be arsed tonight and would much rather be on the sofa with a glass of wine. But needs must. The address is down a country lane, in a charming house that looks like it might be an old barn conversion or something similar. It's a long narrow house with wobbly walls. So, whatever it is that brings Clio some Clarity, she's doing nicely financially out of it. Either that or she has a rich husband. I don't envy anyone with a husband, rich or not. I may not be mega-rich but at least I have my freedom. I park up and knock on the front door.

A woman answers wearing jeans and chequered shirt. She has a layered grey bob, a bit like mine but with a better cut.

'Hi. It's Lucy, isn't it? Come in.'

She sounds almost normal. I mean, she sounds completely normal. I'm so used to meeting weird types with this bootcamp thing, that it's pleasantly surprising to have someone who seems normal.

'Hi, yes, thanks,' I say and step into her hallway. It's a snug place with unrendered walls, so you can see the stonework, which looks like it's been built by hand. The hallway has a nice atmosphere, woolly scarves and duffel coat on hooks, a few pairs of shoes, Crocs and walking boots strewn under the stairs. It smells nice too, not the usual patchouli-type wellness joss sticks or oil burners, just a scent of cleanness and old stone. Clio shows me through to her therapy room. It has pale green walls and a chaise longue that looks really comfortable and I'm hoping I'll be lying down on that because I really could do with a rest. Beside it is a comfortable-looking office chair and along one wall there are shelves of books, a mix of novels and books about psychology and physiology and other 'ologies. There are lots of pot plants in this room, including trays of succulents in all shapes and sizes along the window sill. I have quite a few succulents too at home, as they're really hard to kill. Usually I am the Grim Reaper to most indoor plants.

'You like aeoniums,' I say, nodding towards the window.

'Yes, I love them. Almost impossible to murder.'

'That's what I was thinking! I love the purple ones.'

'Yes, me too, though my favourite is the dinner plate aeonium. Perfect spiral design yet flat as a plate, hence the name. Flowers once then dies. But it's easy to propagate babies from the old one. You should try those. Please, take a seat.'

She gestures for me to sit on the chaise longue. I suddenly realise that amid the madness of this week's work deadlines, I haven't even read the details of what Clarity with Clio is all about, so I listen to her introductory spiel with interest. She sits in her therapist chair with what seems like a genuine smile. It's actually a relief to meet someone in wellness who doesn't immediately feel like an inveterate bullshitter. Then I recall that Tara said her session with Clio was 'life-changing'. That sounds good. Or was Tara just showing off? I guess I'll soon find out.

'Thank you for choosing me as one of your bootcamp four. I often wonder if my sessions sound a bit dull in comparison with such things as magnets being put in unmentionable places.'

I genuinely laugh at that. 'Right?! There was no way I was signing my bum up for that one!'

'Same!' says Clio. 'So, mine is more mundane than any of those newer therapies. Yet I like to think of mine as a deeper experience which will hopefully have more meaning for my clients. Now, have you heard of past-life regression?'

Oh God, yes, it's coming back to me now. It doesn't explain much on the website but past-life regression was mentioned, which I quickly googled and it sounded to me like classic wellness bullshit.

'Only from the spiel about this session, to be honest.'

'I can see by your face that it's a phrase that doesn't appeal to you, perhaps?'

'Well, yes. I've been finding a lot of this wellness stuff to be absolute rubbish.'

'Fair enough,' says Clio. 'The first time I heard of past-life, I thought, what's this arrant nonsense?'

'Ha ha! Exactly!'

'But then, it did change my life. Fundamentally. And forever. So, I'd like to explain a bit more about it first, if that's all right.'

'Of course.' Okay, so I'm hooked now. How is this thing life-changing? Maybe I need a bit of changing of my life these days, who knows? I'm eager to hear more and because Clio is so down-to-earth, I'm not wearing my usual wellness face, which is somewhere between incredulity and sarcasm.

Clio runs her fingers through her hair. I really want mine cut in her style now that I've seen it. It has these bouncy layers that frame her face really well and somehow the shades of white and grey she has really bring out her startling blue eyes. My grey hair just seems to make me look older. I've thought about going back to dyeing it but I really can't be arsed. All that hassle with roots coming through, no thanks. I wish mine brought out the light in my skin and eyes, like hers does. Clio is the epitome of a cooler older woman, about my age, in fact, I'd say fifty-two? But she looks so at ease with herself and so limber, I'd say she could be anything from forty onwards. She's hard to place. There's something enigmatic about her.

'Do feel free to lie down, while I'm explaining this,' she offers and I can't wait. It's Friday evening and I'm so sleepy after a long week. The chaise longue is very nice and smells of lavender or rosemary or something like that. Everything smells nice here. I'm stretched out, my head on what I now realise is a scented pillow and I'm very, very comfortable.

'What we'll be doing this evening, Lucy, is taking a flying visit to one of your past lives. Now, that might sound dreadfully woo-woo and silly. But I promise you, it doesn't matter a jot whether you believe in reincarnation or not. None of that is necessary for this experience to be useful and interesting for you. It's not about what you believe. Some people say it's real, but for others, it's a journey into your subconscious, which is a pretty fascinating place to be, since most of our lives are spent in the front of our heads. Wouldn't it be nice to know what's going on under the bonnet?'

'I've no idea what's going on under my bonnet,' I reply and sigh. 'Just the other day I found myself sobbing in a coffee shop.'

I don't know why I suddenly decided to tell Clio that. But somehow, I knew it'd be okay. Something about her, and her voice, and this room, makes me feel safe yet also energised. I really am not sleepy at all. I'm relaxed but wide awake and fully switched on. I don't think I've felt that way for a long time. And if I do end up telling her stuff, then I never have to see her again, do I? That's the nice thing about a therapist.

'Sorry to hear that, Lucy. Was there something particular that set that off, do you think?'

'Just feeling pretty low about myself, in general. But also there's this . . . sadness, I suppose you'd call it. Just general sadness. And lack of patience with everything, especially work. I think part of it's left over from my father's death seven years ago. I'm usually pretty buoyant about everything. Sarcasm gets me through life quite efficiently. Just lately . . . I don't know. I'm not sure why things are getting on top of me so much recently.'

'I'm hoping that by the end of today's session, the reason might become clearer. So, are you happy to continue?'

'Yeah, sure,' I say. I like the sound of her voice. Let's do this thing. Let's see if it's as life-changing as Tara claimed. If not, it's my last wellness session. I add, 'I'm just glad nobody will be waving anything silly over my body or invoking healing spirits. Unless you are?'

Clio laughs. 'God, no! No hokum, I promise you. There's so much to be interested in within every human brain, that we don't need any gimmicks. Just one human brain connecting with another. Okay, so, I'm going to talk you through a kind of guided journey into your subconscious. It's not hypnosis, so don't worry – I won't be making you bark like a dog or any of that rubbish.'

'Thank God for that!'

'I just have one question. Do you have aphantasia?'

'I've never heard of it, so I doubt it. It sounds like that old Disney flick with the ballet-dancing hippos.'

'Ah, yes, ha ha! That's a classic, *Fantasia*. But this is to do with not having mental images. Some people's brains don't provide them with a mental picture at all. They use movement, direction, kinaesthesia and description to access images mentally instead. Does that sound like you?'

'No, not at all. I can see things in my head all the time. Things I'd rather not see, sometimes.'

Immediately, an image of my dad springs to mind. A moment when he was in a hell of a lot of pain and in the hospice bed and we were all in the room with him. Mum was stoic, while Shirl and I were sobbing. Why did I have to think of that shitty horrible moment right now, when I was feeling so good?

'It can be a curse as well as a gift,' says Clio, again as if she knows my thoughts, or at least could guess the type of content.

'Amen to that,' I say with a sigh. 'But is that really a thing, where some people don't have any mental images? None at all?'

'It is, absolutely,' says Clio. 'Do you have an inner voice, a voice in your head that talks to you and comments on things you're experiencing?'

'Yes, of course. Everybody does.' Then I realise that . . . could it be like this aphantasia? 'You're not telling me some people don't have that?'

'That's right. One term for it is anendophasia. No inner monologue.'

I sit up and look round at Clio. 'You know what, I'd pay good money to have my inner voice removed!'

Clio laughs and replies, 'I know what you mean. Mine can be such a bitch sometimes!'

'Yes!' I agree. 'I'm like, whose side are you on anyway?!'

'So, we know now that you have inner imagery and voice. If you'd like to lie back down, we can begin with closing your eyes.'

I do so and await whatever comes next. I'm actually enjoying this. It doesn't feel like wellness. It just feels like chilling with a really interesting, educated person.

Clio continues, 'If you'd like to close your eyes, then do so, but you don't have to. Another extraordinary thing about our brains is that we can visualise mental images even with our eyes open.'

It's never occurred to me before that I can do this, but I can. How weird is that? Brains are amazing. I look to my top right and, even with my eyes open, I can still visualise a KitKat, just sitting there, waiting to be devoured. Mmmm. Anyway, I must concentrate. I close my eyes and settle down.

'Firstly, you're going to picture yourself at the top of a

staircase. It's a beautiful staircase, not a shabby or unnerving one. It could be sweeping and grand, like one that Scarlett O'Hara might tip-tap down in *Gone with the Wind*.'

Clio has hit the jackpot there with that old movie. One of my dad's favourites.

'Or if you're not familiar with that reference, think of Rose on the stairs in *Titanic*, looking at Jack, ready for adventure.'

Both work for me, to be honest. I always wanted to go to that party in the bowels of the ship and smoke roll-ups and dance reels.

'I know *Gone with the Wind* well,' I say. 'I used to watch old movies with my dad.'

'I remember that about old films and your dad,' says Clio. 'You mentioned it in your questionnaire when you were asked about your favourite childhood memory.'

So I did. I'd forgotten that. Post-menopause brain. I can't remember a damn thing I did from one day to the next. But my long-term memory is sharp as a tack.

'So, Lucy, let's focus,' says Clio, bringing me back to the task in hand. 'The steps are pleasant and well made. When you walk down this staircase you are heading for a place you want to go to. You're eager to go, but let's just slow you down a little, so we don't trip up. Let's take it a step at a time, carefully feeling each foot touch base with each step as you descend, down, down and further down to the bottom of the staircase.'

I can see it all. It's like something from an early Disney princess movie, like *Sleeping Beauty* or *Cinderella* from the fifties. It's ornate and brightly lit and the steps are cool, like marble and I'm barefoot for some reason. As I step downwards, I begin to feel heavier in my body, as if I'm pressing into the chaise longue, but not oppressively, more in a comfortable way, like truly relaxing.

'When you reach the base of the staircase, you see a corridor of many doors before you. It's a long, wide and welcoming corridor that you are keen to go down. You know that those doors are there for you and you alone. This corridor is interesting and has a positive atmosphere to it, one of secrets and adventures ahead. It's an energising, curious place where you absolutely want to be. You're eager to walk down this corridor and try one of these doors and see where it'll take you. Even though you can't see through the doors – none of them have windows – you know deep down that each door does not only lead to a room, but to a place and time far away from where you are now. This galvanises you. You want to choose one and try it. Walk down the corridor now, nice and slowly, no need to rush. You have all the time in the world to make your choice. Think of which one calls to you. One of them feels right. One of them is the one that will take you where you want to go. You can see it now and you're going to stop in front of it and reach out your hand.'

I'm doing it all. The corridor has pale green walls, not white like a hospital. The doors are dark wood, solid and dependable. The fourth one down on the left is calling me. It's just like Clio says. It feels like I absolutely must go there. I approach and put my hand on the door handle and wait. I'm buzzing with excitement. How weird is this! It's just a daydream, just a thought, but I'm desperate to see what's behind that door . . .

'It's time now, Lucy. Time to firmly turn that handle and see what's behind the door. I'm going to wait while you go through and let you take in everything you see. Then, when you're ready, I want you to tell me about it.'

As I turn the handle, I feel it almost vibrating in my hand, as if it's alive. I push the door inward and step through the doorway. I'm immediately backstage at a theatre. The light is dim back here and the atmosphere is hushed. I can hear there is a performance going on and I have to keep quiet. I look down and I'm wearing a white shirt with the cuffs turned up, with brown slacks and brogues and I'm carrying a clipboard. I'm a man, I just know it. I run my fingers through my hair and there's a kind of waxy substance there to keep my hair in place, short back and sides. Backstage is loaded up with props of all kinds like wagon wheels and swords and mirrors. Then a door opens to my right and a gaggle of chorus girls comes out quickly, whispering and fussing with their hair and checking each other's costumes. They're wearing sparkling white outfits with short flowy skirts and pale feathers on their heads. They have exquisitely painted faces and yet look so human in their worry about how they look and whether their headdresses are on straight.

'Where are you now?' comes Clio's voice, but it's as if it comes from another place entirely, not in my mind or in this theatre but somewhere else far away.

'I'm in the theatre, in the wings.'

I describe to Clio everything I can see. She asks about the smells backstage and the sounds coming from the whispering girls and the performers on the stage and textures of the curtains and how my shoes feel on my feet. I can describe everything, it's so ultra-real, like more real than real. I'm absolutely there, in that moment, rich with detail.

'What do you need to do next?' Clio asks.

'I have to get these girls on stage. They're doing the next number. It's a big number, all choreographed and co-ordinated. We've been practising it for months and some of these girls are so unreliable, they're often late or asking for advances on their pay. One I'm looking at now, she fainted with hunger the other night, I remember it. I lent her a few cents to get herself a meal but I doubt I'll ever get it back. This isn't their only job, most of them. They clean hotels or look after rich folks' babies. They're waitresses in shabby cafés or tend bar in a dive on the corner of a forlorn city street. They want to be stars, like the girl on stage now. She's shining with talent and her eyes are dark with stage make-up and her lips deep red. The man beside her is a star too, tall and handsome, hair perfectly slicked back. All the chorus girls want to be with him. For now, though, they have to perform. The guy on stage tries to kiss the girl but she's too shy and flits off to the other side of the stage, while he raises his eyes and the orchestra wakes up and the music swells. He starts to sing a song and then I know I have to get the girls ready to go on. They look to me for their cue and I just know the right moment. "Tits and teeth!" I whisper at them and they titter and giggle as they file onto the stage in perfect symmetry. They're good girls really. They work their arses off.

'I watch the number play out perfectly, as the leading lady comes around to my side and says, "Hardly a goddamned soul in tonight. How are we gonna make it to the end of the week, let alone Christmas?"'

I shrug my shoulders. I know what she means. Everyone here is too poor, after paying for food, rent and heat, to spend their few cents left on a seat at the theatre.

Then I hear Clio's disembodied voice again.

'Where are you? And when are you there? And how do you feel about being there?'

And I know the answer without pause. 'It's 1933 and I'm in a small theatre in New York. I'm the stage manager and I'm responsible for all of these people. They look to me for guidance and I want to tell them it'll all be all right. But I can't. The country is in a depression and nobody has any money for fripperies. The theatre might close down, the manager told me. But despite all this worry, I don't want to be anywhere else. I love my job. I never wanted to be on the stage, the centre of attention. I love organising things behind the scenes. I love making the whole operation come together without having to wear the daft stage make-up and show myself to the public. But even though I love my job, I'm fearful of what might happen to these show folk if we can't get more punters through the door. It's hard being the one they all look to, the face of the management, who hide away in their offices. Meanwhile, I keep everything running. I'm not famous, I'm not recognisable, but I'm essential.'

I watch the girls doing their number, feathers swaying, suffused with the smells of sweat and shoe polish and old dusty drapes. I've never felt more present in my life. I can feel my flat chest beneath my shirt rising and falling as I breathe, feel the appendage between my legs that is partly sticking to my thigh in the heat here in the theatre, taking in how strange it is to be a man and yet feeling utterly secure in the knowledge that I am a man. 'I am a stage manager in 1930s New York and my name is Frank.'

There's still a part of me that absolutely knows that – physically – I'm lying on a chaise longue in a barn conversion in Langton Green. But my mind is in another place entirely.

'You're going to leave the stage now, Frank,' says Clio's voice. But I'm reluctant to go. I need to make sure the girls come off quickly for the next number, because the guy playing the gangster always starts his dialogue too soon and it's scrappy.

'You're going to go back to that door where you entered this place and open it. Then you're going to leave and enter the corridor again.'

I want to stay. But I have to obey Clio's voice too, as it's in control, somehow. I do as she says and I walk away from the stage. The song the leading man is crooning grows faint as I head for the door I came through, my brown slacks huffing as I stride along, my leather shoes creaking. I open the door and I go through it.

'I'm in the corridor,' I say. 'I'm a woman again and I'm wearing the thick woollen leggings and corduroy skirt I came in. And I'm me again. I'm just . . . me.'

'Good. Well done, Lucy. Open your eyes now.'

I don't want to. I want to be back in that theatre in 1933. But I can't. It's gone now. It feels like it's gone forever. I open my eyes.

Chapter 10

'Can you sit up for me, Lucy?' says Clio's soothing voice.

I do so and I feel a little strange, a little light-headed. Clio is leaning over and passing me a glass of water. I drink it, gladly. Just water, normal tap water, not some dumb smoothie or juice cleanse. I need it. My mouth is dry as sandpaper. Clio sits silently and waits.

'Wow!' I say, now feeling refreshed and more normal. 'I just . . . I can't believe that. That was . . . I don't even know how to describe it.'

'You described it beautifully,' said Clio. 'You gave such exquisite detail.'

'That's because I could smell, feel, see, hear everything. Everything. What . . . what does it all mean?'

Clio smiles and leans forward, her elbows on her knees, her hands clasped beneath her chin.

'What do you think it means, Lucy?'

'I don't know. I don't know who Frank is.'

'Frank is a man with a lot of responsibility,' says Clio. I

look at her and somehow, even with my eyes open, I'm seeing out of Frank's eyes again.

'He is,' I mutter.

'A lot of people rely on him. They look to him for guidance. He's alone there, in the wings. He doesn't want to be a performer. He doesn't want the limelight like they do. He wants to make change in the background, where he can do some good. But it's pretty hard being that person, the way they all look up to him. The way they want to know from him, is everything going to be okay? But he can't answer that. He's a leader and he's responsible for them. But he's alone. He loves his role but it's not easy. Does that sound familiar, Lucy?'

It does sound horribly familiar. She could be describing me, at Beane & Co. The responsibility of management is what I always craved, climbing my way to the top. But now I'm there, or nearly there, it's the responsibility for others that wears me down. I want to go beyond that, I want to be making the business better, behind the scenes, away from the limelight.

'My God, it's me. It's me, Clio. It's how I am at work. It's the promotion I want, to get away from being responsible for all those people.'

'That's marvellous,' says Clio, smiling broadly. 'Clever brain. Clever you!'

'But . . . but why the 1930s? I mean, I love history, but usually it's medieval stuff, or the Tudors, that kind of history. I've never thought about that time period before.'

'Are you sure about that?' Clio says, gently.

And suddenly, for the second time tonight, I'm transported to the sofa with my dad. I'm seven years old, and we're watching old black-and-white movies about theatre folk, with elaborate dance numbers peopled by dozens of chorus girls, choreographed by Busby Berkeley, one of my dad's favourites.

'It's my dad and me!' I cry. 'On the sofa, watching old movies. I know all the old movies. If you're ever doing a pub quiz and movies come up, I'm your gal!'

'I'll bear that in mind!' says Clio. 'Clever you,' she adds again. 'Your mind took you exactly where it needed to go. Have you been thinking a lot about work lately, and about your dad?'

'Oh blimey, so much!' I say. And I tell Clio everything about the last few weeks, about my sister and mum hassling me to move to New Zealand, about the promotion at work. I'm about to slag off my rival Tara, when I suddenly remember she's been here and seen Clio too. That riles me up immeasurably. I'm so mad that Tara Harryman has been here too: here, this special place with this special person that I've just discovered. Urgh, it feels like I can't have anything without that Tara woman trying to stick her oar in.

'Where are you now, Lucy? Not here, that's for sure.'

I'm dragged back to reality. Clio's voice is calm, pleasant, not stressy. I rarely hear voices like that in my life, not at work, or in my family.

'Sorry,' I say and grin nervously. I don't want to tell her about Tara, but also I do. I wish I could. But I have to stay professional.

'Nothing to be sorry for. That's our time more or less up now, Lucy.'

Oh no! I'm actually shattered but I don't want this session to end. It's been . . . magical.

'Do you have any questions for me?' Clio asks.

'Yes . . . I . . . I don't really understand what happened tonight. I guess it was a trip into my subconscious. But is it a past life? Was I Frank once? Was that me?'

Clio smiles again and tips her head slightly to the side. 'What do *you* think?'

'The cynic in me says no. I don't believe in all that bullshit! But it felt so real. So utterly . . . other, from my usual life.'

'Perhaps instead of worrying about how real it is, or not, or whether reincarnation exists or not, perhaps instead we can simply marvel at the wonder of the subconscious, at the complexity of the human brain. And perhaps that in itself is enough.'

Clio stands and I know it's time to go, but I don't want it to be. I want to talk to her about the complexity of the human brain. And many other things.

When we reach her front door, I say, 'Thank you, Clio. I don't know if you've restored my faith in wellness culture, because I feel like you're offering something different, something so much richer than the vagaries of that messed-up wellness industrial complex. I feel like you give people access to something really important.'

'Thank you, Lucy. Those are kind and generous words. I'm glad you enjoyed our session and hope you've enjoyed the whole experience of the wellness bootcamp.'

'Not really!' I say, laughing. 'But tonight was great.'

Clio thanks me again and sees me out to my car and off I go home, driving through the dark streets, frost already twinkling on the roadside vegetation on this cold January night. I can't stop thinking about that session. It was the last thing I expected to happen, that anything in this wellness nonsense could have moved me so much and engaged me so completely. Begrudgingly, I realise that Tara was absolutely right about Clarity with Clio. It is life-changing. Maybe this is one thing that Tara and I can agree on.

I've just realised that, even though I moaned about this bootcamp (which is a total misnomer by the way – sitting in four different rooms over four Fridays with essential oils and juice drinks and comfy chairs isn't exactly like yomping with the Paras), I'm actually going to miss doing it. Not because the other three wellness types were anything I'm going to take seriously. Not in the slightest! But they were at least entertaining. And they did at least make a change from the sofa and takeaway of my usual Friday night. But this session with Clio . . . this was something quite different. Something beyond the entertainment of the others . . . something deeper. I've never had an experience quite like it. I've had dreams at night, of course. I've had daydreams too, like we all do. This was something apart from those everyday experiences. This gave me access to a part of my brain I feel cut off from. Some kind of willing subconscious that opened up to me simply because Clio wanted it to. This isn't on the same plane as vapes and fossils and ice baths. This is something quite extraordinary. Years ago, as a young woman, I went flying in a light aircraft with an old pilot boyfriend. I was terrified for the first ten minutes or so. I wouldn't even look out of the window. Then, once I opened my eyes and realised how beautiful it was, I loved every minute. When we touched down again on the runway, I shouted, 'Again! Again!' Flying was nothing like how I thought it would be. I was surprised by joy. That reminds me of tonight. I walked into Clio's room tonight expecting another bit of nonsense.

But I left it suffused with something akin to wonder. And I want more of that.

So much so, that once I'm home after Clio's session, I decide to send her an email asking for another session. Of all four, hers is the one that not only feels most useful but also doesn't seem to have a hint of a grift about it. Have I actually found the Holy Grail of wellness, the therapist who actually helps people? It certainly feels that way. No hard sell, no bullshit. Just a relaxing yet wonderfully powerful experience that I'm dead keen to try again. She replies soon after and sends me to her online booking form. There's a payment page and on there is an option to donate to two cancer charities to support people with their treatment. That's a surprise. I wonder what Clio's connection is to cancer, if any. Of course, largely because of Dad, I donate fifty pounds to each of the cancer charities. I even feel a bit righteous, helping others. Fifty pounds is probably a drop in the ocean for what people need but it's something and I'm happy to do it. It's a great idea to put that on there and just proves again how much I'm beginning to admire Clio. I've booked another appointment with her for the same time next week and honestly, I can't bloody wait.

Still reeling from the session with Clio, I meet up with Jacqui for dinner out a few days later in one of our favourite cosy, little bistros and I cannot wait to tell her all about it. I recount the whole thing, in precise detail and what strikes me as I'm telling it is that I can remember every nuance of that experience – especially the 1933 part – and yet in my everyday brain-fogged memory-challenged life I struggle to remember if I have my trousers on the right way round.

'That's amazing!' says Jacqui, as she polishes off her steak frites, while I've been talking so much my dish is still eighty per cent full of spaghetti vongole. 'Particularly considering the other three sessions were so silly.'

'Well, you see, that's the interesting thing. I think there's more to this wellness stuff than meets the eye. I got something out of all of them, even if it was just someone being nice to me for an hour. But this one with Clio was something else. It felt . . . profound, you know?'

'It sounds more like psychotherapy or a version of it, than a wellness activity as such,' Jacqui ponders. 'It's been dressed up as past-life regression to make it sound more fancy. And maybe it attracts more vulnerable people because they are more attracted to wonder-drug one-size-fits-all types of therapies.'

'I agree with you, that most of what these wellness types tell you is rubbish. But, in this case, Clio was really clear that it didn't matter whether you believe in past-life regression or not, as it's more about what's going on in your subconscious and that's helpful anyway. It was much, *much* better than the other three wellness sessions. It made me think a lot about my dad and his effect on my life. And also how I feel about my job. I wasn't expecting that at all.'

Jacqui is nodding and listening hard, with her eyes narrowed, flicking away her brown and golden highlighted fringe as if that helps her listen better, her fingers playing with the end of a plait tossed over her shoulder. 'Look, this stuff is really interesting. I mean, I know you never meant to do any of this wellness thing but it's actually turned out rather fascinating. What is it that you meant about getting something out of all of these sessions? What is it that the four sessions had in common?'

She's in journalist mode, I can tell. But I don't mind, I can't stop thinking about all this wellness stuff these days. It always helps me think straight to throw ideas about with Jacqui. She has such a great brain.

'It's something about someone being devoted to you and you alone for an hour or however long. How often do any of us get that in the rest of our lives?'

'Very true,' says Jacqui and rolls her eyes. 'The last time Barna gave me a shoulder massage was on our second date, I think. Around about sixteen years ago!'

'Right?! Same for most people, I'd imagine. As bizarre as all this wellness therapy stuff is, something that's all about love doesn't sound so bad – even if it is as batshit as this. But . . . only if it's genuine. And paying someone to direct loving energy into you is appealing . . . but of course it's not as nice as someone choosing to love you and wanting to spend time with you.'

'Well, yeah, lots of people will pay a shitload to feel like that.'

I'm on a roll now. Ideas are coming thick and fast. 'It's big business, loneliness. Plus, it's not just that, it's not just about human contact and the illusion of someone caring for you. I'm really intrigued by something Yorick said to me, about the child and the old woman, the wise old ways and this kind of . . . well, I suppose you could call it the upstart science of western medicine. It's not been around long!'

'Yeah, that sounds like it makes sense,' replies Jacqui. 'But ancient medicine wasn't all that reliable either. There were many dangerous practices in primitive medicine that killed people. Just look at the four humours and all that nonsense old-timey doctors used to believe in. Think how many people died due to lack of antiseptic conditions in surgery and childbirth, or from lack of antibiotics with infections. You can't just say that all ancient medicine is wise and the new stuff is bollocks. Science doesn't have all the answers but it's a damn sight more reliable than this woo-woo stuff.'

'But I think those examples you gave were all on the pretence of science, even though we know now it was nonsense. I'm talking about really ancient stuff, like from thousands of years ago. Stuff we might've forgotten. Maybe there's something to it?'

Jacqui's really activated by this too now, leaning over the table as I try to shovel in forkfuls of spaghetti every time she speaks – I'm starving. 'Don't you think though that this is one of the main things the wellness industry plays on? Ancient equals good. Modern equals bad. Surely that's too simplistic a way of looking at our health. But that's how this industry works: a bunch of tropes it wheels out every time. Ancient wisdom . . . making out that optimising yourself makes you a better person . . . creating a mystique around it all by saying these are secrets that are being kept from you. It starts to overlap with conspiracy theories in that way . . . Lu, this is really, really great stuff. I want to write about it!'

'Then, you should! What are you thinking, an article?'

Jacqui is lit up like a Christmas tree. It's so good to see her like this about something. She's been so fed up lately with her editor giving her the dullest of dull stories. I think she'd be brilliant if she wrote about this topic.

'A series of articles, I'd say. There are loads of local wellness businesses around here. I could interview them plus you, or you can be an anonymous source, if you like.'

'Oh, yes please. I have to keep up the pretence for work about all this wellness shite. I'll be "deep background", if that's what they call it. Just call me Deep Throat from *All the President's Men*!'

'I'm not calling you Deep Throat.'

'Oh, go on!'

'Listen, a series of articles about the wellness industry – like the whole industrial complex of it and what are the issues involved with alternative medicine or wellness practices not proven by science. And . . . and . . .'

'Get your notebook out!' I cry, as I'm shovelling in more pasta. 'You know what you're like. You go off on one and forget it all the next day because your memory is almost as shit as mine.'

Jacquie scrabbles around in her voluminous mum-type handbag and finds a notebook and pen and starts writing away like mad. I'm so happy to see her excited about a new idea. I'm so mad at her stupid boss for his constant rejections; maybe he'll like this one. And if I can help her at all, I feel better because she is such a huge help to me, I often worry there's an imbalance in our relationship, as I'm always moaning and she's always listening. I couldn't cope without her, I honestly could not. It's a joy to watch her scribbling away and it gives me a chance to get on with my bloody dinner. Totally my fault. I talk too damn much (or so Martin used to tell me, often).

'Okay,' Jacqui says, coming up for air, while I finally finish my cold clams and spaghetti. 'The big questions I have so far are as follows. Look read it here.'

She turns her notebook round and shoves it at me.

WELLNESS BOLLOCKS ARTICLE
- Does any of it actually work?
- If it does work, is it just the placebo effect?
- Do these wellness people believe in what they're doing? Or do they know it's all a grift?
- The wellness industry has a lot wrong with it – too many scammers and too much snake oil, preying on vulnerable people desperate for help, especially women – but also there are surprising benefits that somehow rise above the bullshit.
- Could wellness actually be the latest way to make women feel shit about themselves, i.e. if you're not 'optimising' your wellness, then it's just another thing you're failing at, bitch.

I laugh at that and hand it back to her.

'This is brilliant,' I tell her. 'You're brilliant. You must do it.'

'I think I will! It'll be fun to work with you on it too, chick, plus because I'll be researching it all, I could send you some stuff to help you with your wellness speech at the staff conference.'

'Ah, that would be great! That's a deal.'

I raise my glass and she reciprocates.

Jacqui makes the toast: 'Two old mates taking down the wellness industry, one wanker at a time.'

Chapter 11

I get through the next few days buoyed by the tonic of seeing how excited Jacqui is about her new story. I haven't seen her like that in a long time. And, to be honest, I haven't been this excited about anything for years, not even when Jacqui went to Japan on holiday and brought me back a selection box of KitKat varieties. Now, that was pretty damn exciting. But surpassing even that is my anticipation of the next session with Clio. I can't get over how weird and wonderful it felt to enter my subconscious in such an unusual way. I mean, we all have dreams, some more than others. Mine are generally about ennui and anxiety. If I'm not trapped inside a filing cabinet, I've lost my handbag in a foreign country. This was something quite different. I don't believe in past lives BUT being in Frank's head and shoes was an experience I've never had, not even in a dream. Where the hell did that come from? Why did my brain decide to put that world behind that door? It's blown my mind. I don't know how it works but I want to do it again.

The night before my next session with Clio I can barely sleep, as I'm buzzing about going there again. I feel like a teenager going on a first date! I don't fancy Clio, if that's what you're wondering. It's not like that with me. I'm not really interested in that side of things, not interested in crushes or sex or any of that stuff, whoever it may be. But I am very drawn to Clio and I don't know why. Making a new connection with someone – even if you're paying them – is a bit thrilling, and it's been so long since I've felt this way about meeting someone new. I'm beginning to wonder if maybe Clio finds me interesting too, after all, I'm not a boring person, or at least I hope I'm not. And I bet Clio has some ultra dull clients she can't want to get rid of. Maybe Clio is looking forward to my next session too, who knows! Something about our connection feels deeply personal and special. But I am getting ahead of myself, I know that. I'm not a fool. I'm just one of many clients to her. It's just that I don't make connections very often. When I do, they go deep, very deep. Like with my dad, with Jacqui, even with Martin (until it all went to shit). I don't let people in easily. It takes a gargantuan effort. I just don't trust people, really. So when I find someone I feel I can trust (which is hardly ever), I go all in.

Finally, Friday evening arrives and I drive with a big grin on my face to Clio's house. She greets me and seems genuinely happy to see me too.

'I feel so comfortable here,' I say to Clio. I'm not one for professions of emotion, except to my closest people – well, basically, only Jacqui, now Dad's gone. So this is unusual for me. 'When I lie down on this chaise longue, it feels like I've been here a dozen times, not just once.'

'That's wonderful to hear!' says Clio, tonight in brown

125

cords, slipper socks and a chunky cream Fair Isle jumper. She's one of those people who are effortlessly cool, like Jacqui. It'd make you sick if you didn't like them already. 'How did you feel after last week's appointment?'

'Honestly it just blew me away. I couldn't stop thinking about it. About Frank, and old movies, and how it seemed to represent a part of me, my work self. And also reminded me so much of being with my dad. It really moved me. It's been on my mind all week.'

'That's fascinating,' says Clio. 'Was it comforting, to be reminded of your dad that way?'

'Yeah, it was. It wasn't him, of course. Frank is nothing like my dad. Frank was me, somehow. But just to be in that world. To see it writ large in my mind's eye, instead of living in this little black and white square on a telly in the seventies . . . that was extraordinary.'

'That's a good step, that you recognise Frank is yourself. Have you been thinking about him this week? And have you been thinking about your father? I can tell you two had a profoundly special relationship. But what did you think of Frank, of being Frank?'

'Yeah, his situation really resonated with me. I felt the weight of responsibility on his shoulders, for all the staff he's in charge of, for their performance but also their future, their happiness. It's very familiar to me. Also, it was funny to think how odd it was to be a man, and in that place. The whole atmosphere of that theatre backstage. It was so *real*. And just sitting there waiting for my brain to reveal it. If I hadn't opened that door, would it have been a different place, time and person? Or was the whole thing my brain just making it up on the fly? Screening improvised movies in the first person at a moment's notice? Whatever it was, it was pretty awe-inspiring. I'd like to experience it again and see where my brain goes this time.'

Clio is pleased, I can tell. She's smiling broadly and nodding her head to each point I make.

'These are great questions to ask,' she says. 'And I'd love to discuss all those questions with you. But I'm also aware of the time we have and I want you to spend as much time in your altered state as possible. I call it an altered state because it's a bland enough term to mean anything to anyone. It's a past life if you want it to be or it's a trip to your subconscious instead, whatever you prefer. So, shall we make a start?'

She goes through the same process as last time, the stairs, the corridor. I've latched onto the tenth door on the right. I wanted to go further down the corridor this time, as it felt like I'd be going deeper into my subconscious.

'Are you ready to go in?' says Clio's voice. It already feels very far away from me. I've passed over into a new place. It's the weirdest thing.

'Yes,' I answer, excited to go through.

I open the door.

The first thing that hits me is the sun in my eyes.

I squint and I can feel the warmth of the sun . . . and that the air is British, that I'm not abroad. I don't know how I know that, I just do. It feels like British air! You know when you go on holiday overseas and you step off the plane and the air feels different, like cooler in Prague or thicker in Rome. The air here has the warmth of an early British summer, like May kind of time, I think.

'Tell me everything,' says Clio.

I take a step forward and I'm on a grassy hill; my muscles

can feel that's the position we're in. I've moved my gaze and I can see clearly now.

'I'm in a field on a steep slope, coming down it to a rutty pebble-strewn path that leads off between two hedgerows. I know the way to go. My feet are taking me there. I'm walking along the path and through the hedgerows on either side I can see farmer's fields with growing crops in them.'

I carry on describing everything to Clio as I go. I'm looking at the crops and they're so pretty. I think it's wheat; it's quite tall and a kind of glaucous blue, that lovely green-blue that early wheat can have. I feel like this place is very, very familiar. It's kind of spooking me, to be honest. Last time, everything was unfamiliar, in that I'd never been to that place, though it was familiar from the old movies Dad and I watched, of course. But this place . . . it feels like I've been here in a dream before. Have you ever had that? When you're dreaming at night and you just know you've been there before, but only in dreams? This isn't like that though. I think I've been here in real life, a very long time ago. I can see at the end of this shadowed path, where the hedgerows throw dappled light across its winding way, that there is an opening into another place. This path has been made by human feet, I can tell, tramping through this shortcut for centuries. They call them desire paths, don't they? I read that once. Lovely phrase. And I can feel the history shivers of all of those many, many thousands of Britons that have tramped down this path in all that time, almost as if they're walking beside me. I'm eager to get to that opening at the end. I know that when I reach there, I will see a place I remember, but for now it's on the tip of my tongue, at the edge of my inner vision, just out of reach.

I'm there and there's a twist in the path, heading down

now, hard-baked mud steps with sprouts of grass, leading down and around a bend, so I can't see the end. Oh God, I know these steps so well, it's freaking me out now. Where am I? *When* am I? Will I be surrounded by Saxons and Celts when I get to the bottom? Or Tudors or Georgians? I go faster. I can't wait.

And here I am, at the bottom of the steps, crossing over into another small field, surrounded by trees and there before me is a place I know so well, I want to cry. There's a river running through it, a wooden bridge arching over it, a simple bridge, small and plainly made. It's just as I remember it, where I once stood and dangled jam jars off with string tied around their necks to lower them down into the water and catch minnows and tadpoles. I can't believe I'm here. I'm deep in the Kent countryside and it's the mid-1970s. My heart fills with nostalgia and gratitude that my brain has let me come here again. This is not a past life. This is my life but in my own past. I'm walking over the field towards the water and I'm looking up and down the field, over the bridge to the bright yellow rapeseed field on the other side, looking through the trees to see . . . if he's there . . . if my dad is coming. This was the place he took me and my sister when my mum wanted us out of the house. She'd be cleaning or cooking or on her sewing machine or just in one of her dark moods and she'd say, 'Bert, get these kids out from under my feet, for God's sake.' And he'd say, 'All right, Marge, no need to fret.' Albert and Marjorie, my mum and dad, unhappily married for all the years I knew them. Maybe they were happy once, before we came. That's what I imagined, that my sister and I had ruined their lives, especially my mum's. And especially me, because I'm the eldest. Dad never made me feel like that though. He'd take me and Shirl and bundle us into the car, one of those old Morris Minor Travellers half made of wood. I used to wish we had a dog in the back with us to sprawl about with and chase when we got there but Dad was allergic to dogs and Mum didn't like cats, so we never had them. We had a tortoise for a while called Shelley Winters (loved her in *The Poseidon Adventure* plus she was gorgeous and a bit podgy, which made me feel better about my own podginess, especially since my sister was always stick thin, like Mum). But Shelley the tortoise died during his hibernation. (Yeah, he was a boy called Shelley Winters.) He went to sleep in a cardboard box and never woke up. Good way to go, to be honest.

But Dad isn't here. It's just me, alone. I mount the bridge and walk to the middle. I'm small. I have to climb up onto the bridge's struts to lean over the side. I realise I'm a child. I hadn't realised that yet. I was so caught up with the environment I hadn't noticed my red Clarks shoes – my God, I still wear Clarks today! – with the leaf-shaped cutouts of the red leather. I'm wearing a pinafore dress, red cotton, with short white sleeves. How I loved this dress! White pelerine socks with the patterned little holes all over them. I loved those socks too. I lean over the wooden side of the bridge and stare down into the fast-moving river below. It's rushing along, the sun glinting on its rapid curves and dips, tiny dark fish shooting about and the flash of something larger, a brown trout, I think. The sound of that babbling brook is the most beautiful thing I've heard in years. It's pure and perfect and utterly itself, minding its own business. I am so happy to be here. But also, I feel so alone. I feel very small. Where is everyone?

'Who should be there?' I hear Clio's voice from far away, after describing all this to her.

'Dad. My dad. And Shirl.'

'Then let them find you,' says Clio, mysteriously.

I'm wondering what she means when I feel two hands on my shoulders. Broad hands, holding me steady.

'Don't lean over too far, you daft apeth.'

Oh crikey, I can't believe it. I feel those broad, safe hands easing me down and helping me hop off the bridge's strut to land on my feet and look up.

My dad. My dad!

He's young, so young. It breaks my heart to see him so limber and healthy, when the last time I saw him he was seventy-six, but looked so much older, just before he died. I know he's thirty-five now, because I'm five, I just know that too. He was so handsome, it takes your breath away. Like a young Alan Bates, dark-eyed and cheeky. I can't stop staring at him. Christ, I want to cry my eyes out. But also I'm just so overwhelmed with happiness and love, I can't stop smiling.

'What's all this grinning about, Lu-Lu? You done a secret fart and frightened the fishes?'

I belly-laugh and he does too. He'd never dare say a word like 'fart' at home, in front of Mum. She'd tear a strip off him.

Mum. Is she here? I glance around for her, see if she's carrying my sister on her hip. Shirl is always on my mum's hip, won't leave her alone. I can't see them. And I'm happy I can't see them, if I'm totally honest with myself.

'Where's Shirl and Mum?'

'Home,' says Dad. 'Don't you remember? Shirl's got a sniffle and Mum says she's too little at only two to be gallivanting

131

in the countryside when she's got a sniffle. You've got the memory of a goldfish, you!'

I laugh and say, 'I forgot.' Then, I do a guilty little grin and say, 'I'm glad they're home.'

'Don't you miss your baby sister?' says Dad, smiling. But I know he knows I much prefer it when it's just me and him. I love my sister, I really do. I'm terribly protective of her. But my five-year-old self finds minding her all the time a bit of a trial. And it's nice to have some Saturday time alone with Dad, in our favourite place.

'Jam jars?' I say.

'Not today,' says Dad. 'I forgot. Let's go wading in the shallows and see if we can't catch some naughty minnows in our hands, shall we? Or maybe a spiny stickleback or two. Come on, slowcoach!'

Dad trots off over the bridge and round the side, as I chase him and struggle to keep up. He's got his sandals off already and he's rolling his khaki trouser legs up his hairy calves. I sit down on the grass with a thump on my bottom, thinking if I get grass stains on my special dress, Mum might really kill me this time. I struggle to undo the buckles so Dad comes to help me, pulling off my shoes and socks. Mum's taught me to pop my socks inside my shoes when I take them off but Dad tosses them in the air so they land willy-nilly on the grass. He grasps my hand and leads me down to the water's edge. I'm not afraid the water will be cold. It's a warm day and actually it'll be refreshing to have the cool water undulating over my feet. But there's that sludgy muddy bit on the shore where your feet can sink and you can get stuck and I'm afraid of that. I saw quicksand on telly once and I couldn't get it out of my head, being sucked under and drowning in wet sand or thick mud. Terrified me. So I step gingerly into the shallows, while Dad strides on into the deeper bit of the stream, pulling me onwards, so my feet don't get a chance to sink. We stand in the fast-flowing stream, the water up to just below my knees. Dad hoists up my skirt and tucks it in my knickers. I'm glad because if I get my special dress wet and muddy, Mum will definitely murder me.

Dad's still holding my hand to keep me safe in the flow of water and he says, 'Let's try some one-handed fishing, shall we?'

We both lean down and put our hands in the water. The coolness is lovely, the stream translucent and shadowy, flowing mellifluously across my fingers as they play in the water. I can't see any fishies or tadpoles, but I don't mind. I just love the feel of the water. It's always my favourite thing at school, when they get the water tray out, with the little water wheel in it and the cups. I love baths too, long baths with Matey Bubble Bath – I can't believe they still make that, all these years later. I saw it in Sainsbury's the other day.

Then suddenly, as if the thought of Matey Bubble Bath on a Sainsbury's shelf in 2025 has broken the spell, I hear Clio's voice.

'You're going to come out of the water now, Lucy.'

'No,' I say, defiantly. It's not me talking, but at the same time it is. It's little me. It's little Lu-Lu from the 1970s. She doesn't want to come out of the water. And neither does old Lu either. I squeeze Dad's hand harder and look up at him.

'Time to go, Loopy-Lu,' he says and smiles sadly at me.

'No!' I cry. I can feel hot tears of frustration tipping down my cheeks. 'I won't!'

Then I hear a sound like a whip cracking. I'm scared. I

start and look for reassurance at Dad but realise the noise came from him somehow. He has his other hand up and he's put his thumb and middle finger together.

'Time to go,' he says, but it's Clio's voice too, both together, like a two-part harmony. And he clicks his fingers again and everything goes dark.

The next thing I know, I'm in that corridor again and my hand is on the door handle, and despite wanting to run back into that childhood world as swiftly as my little legs will carry me, I can't do it, as I have no control over my body. My hand pulls the door to and shuts it. I can see by my height that I'm my adult self again, wearing the baggy M&S jeans I came in. But my feet are still wet and I can feel the squelch of mud between my toes.

Chapter 12

My God, how I sob when I open my eyes. It all comes flooding out. I haven't cried like this in years. Clio hands me a box of tissues she has ready on the table – maybe lots of her clients have cathartic sobbing sessions like this. She waits patiently. Eventually, I pull myself together and say sorry.

'No need to apologise. No need at all,' says Clio.

'I wasn't prepared for that, to be honest. I thought in my second session I might go somewhere historical and glamorous, like a jester at the Plantagenet court or being Cleopatra's handmaiden or something. I can't believe I went back to the bridge and saw Dad.'

I sob again. Eventually I pull myself together.

I say, 'He was so young, so beautiful.'

'Do you mind me asking when you lost him?'

'Seven years ago.'

'You said in your medical questionnaire it was lung cancer.'

'Yes, that's right. Awful disease. Dreadful.'

I shudder to think of it. The juxtaposition – of the ravaged man I saw last fading away in a hospice bed and the young, vital chap who minutes ago was rolling up his trouser legs – is shocking.

'I'm so sorry, Lucy.'

'It's all right.'

But it's not all right and we both know that. Clio sits quietly as I gather my thoughts.

'God, Clio, it was so real. He was so real! I can't deal with it.'

I feel breathless and panicky. I can't believe I'm not on hallucinogenic drugs or something. How my mind managed to conjure up something so true to life astonishes me. And it disturbs me.

'Focus on your breathing, Lucy. Slow it down. Count the long length of each breath. One . . . two . . . three . . . '

I've had a few panic attacks in my teens and twenties, but not for decades. I remember now what to do and Clio helps me. Eventually I get it under control and feel less weird.

'We can stop the session now, if you like, Lucy. We only have fifteen minutes left anyway. I actually ended your vision early to discuss the questions we mentioned earlier. But we don't have to talk at all. You can sit quietly and breathe. I'll see you out to your car when you're ready or I can call someone for you to come and stay with you.'

'No, it's okay. I'll be okay. Thank you. Have you got another session after mine?'

'Yes, in a half-hour. I always leave a fifteen-minute break between.'

I'm truly back in reality now. Time has intervened. I feel better and yet worse.

Clio asks, 'Would you like to talk or have a rest for a bit?'

'Talking is okay. I want to talk.'

'Do you want to talk about your dad?'

'Yes, always,' I say and give a hollow laugh. 'He was my best friend. That might sound weird or even pathetic. I don't care really. It's true. Nobody else ever "got" me the way my dad did, except my best friend Jacqui. But it was different, because he was part of me, of course. Blood and bone. He used to say that sometimes: "I love you blood and bone." It's a bit of a shocking thing to say somehow but it's also very powerful. He told me his grandma used to say it to him. He never bothered me, never tried to push me this way or that in my life. He was just proud of me whatever I did. And he was always there to talk to. And I'm still so angry about how he died. He didn't go to the doctor for ages because he hated going to the doctor. He had a cough for months. Nothing made it better. And when he finally did go to his GP, they said it was asthma and gave him an inhaler. That didn't work, then he went back and they said it was an infection and gave him antibiotics. That happened four times – four rounds of antibiotics and words like bronchitis and pneumonia thrown around. He'd stopped smoking in his sixties but not once did any doctor ask him about his smoking. I had to go with him in the end, to the GP, to insist somebody did more tests. That GP actually said to me it might help if he lost weight. Losing weight! For lung cancer! I told them he'd already lost quite a lot of weight, and if he'd had the same GP each time instead of seeing different ones, they'd have noticed that, or at least someone should be weighing him. Not once did they offer an X-ray or biopsy, not until I insisted. And then, lo and behold, lung cancer, stage four. They gave him chemotherapy at Maidstone Hospital.

At the Charles Dickens Day Unit. I always wondered why you'd name a deadly disease after a novelist. Weird. Anyway, the chemo didn't work. He went downhill quickly and into the hospice. I was raging about it.'

'I think you still carry a lot of anger about it.'

'I haven't had a rant like that about my dad's medical care for a while. I realise I still have so much anger about it. It's never really gone away.'

'What other emotions come to mind when thinking about your dad's cancer?'

'Fear.' I don't even know where that word came from. I've shocked myself.

'Fear of what?'

I have to think because I never expected to say that word. 'Fear . . . because . . . it might happen to me. I used to smoke quite a bit. Dad and I smoked together. I hate myself for that, for encouraging him. I should've stopped him. Plus my mum's mum had cervical cancer. She died of that too in dreadful pain, apparently. Or so Mum told us when we were young, too young to hear it really. Gave me nightmares. I never met her, as she died before I was born. Died young. So I've got cancer on both sides of the family. Double whammy. So yeah, I do fear that I'll get cancer too, somewhere in my body. I hadn't realised how much I fear it until I've just said it to you, now.'

Clio pours me a glass of water and I drink it. She seems to intuit that I need refreshment after that revelation. We sit quietly while I drink it and it's not even awkward.

Then Clio says, 'I have something about myself I'd like to share with you. I would never usually do this with clients but I feel like I can trust you, if that's okay with you, Lucy?'

Of course it's okay with me! She's a very intriguing person and I'd love to hear more about her. And I feel really privileged that she trusts me too.

'Lucy, I was diagnosed with cervical cancer too, a few years ago.'

'Oh no!' I cry. I feel desperately sorry for her but also panicky. I realise that even though I've only met this person twice, the thought of her not being around for much longer fills me with fear again. 'Clio, I'm so sorry to hear that. How are you now?'

'I'm absolutely fine, Lucy. Please don't worry. I had surgery to remove the cervix and then started chemotherapy. I was at the Charles Dickens centre at Maidstone too. I used to think the same thing about why they named it after him!'

I add, 'I even looked up if he died of cancer but he didn't. He had a stroke!'

'That makes no sense!' she says and we both laugh, even though the subject matter is grim.

'God, I'm sorry, I interrupted. Please go on.'

'It's fine, Lucy. We have to be able to laugh about these things. But listen, the reason I wanted to share this with you is because of what happened with my treatment. The chemo I had made me feel worse than the cancer itself. So, I decided to stop the chemo very soon after it started. All my doctors argued against it but I was determined. I learnt about past life regression and some other techniques, body movement exercises and thought experiments, in order to cope psychologically with what was happening to my body. And as for my physical health, I devised a whole food diet and other wholesale nutritional changes and soon, the cancer went into remission, amazing all of my doctors.'

'That *is* amazing!' I say and I'm incredibly relieved. And fascinated. 'And so brave to go against the doctors' advice.'

'Well, I would never claim to cure cancer with my therapy – that'd be ridiculous. But I know that I'd be dead if I hadn't stopped that chemo and cleared out my system of all that poison. If all modern medicine can do is poison you to somehow make you better, and our bodies are perfectly designed for us to heal ourselves, then why the hell are we trusting modern medicine with everything? After all, it only became the norm after germ theory was discovered in the nineteenth century. Since then, modern medicine has set its stall out – and I mean that literally; it was just another business like any other, before the NHS, in opposition to so-called quackery. But who decided what was best for our bodies? And how did we get lost along the way? Doctors these days mostly treat us like unruly children.'

'I know that feeling. It used to drive me insane the way some doctors talked to Dad. Like he was a cretin. *He can hear you, you know*, I used to rant at some of them. It drove me nuts.'

Clio nodded her head with her eyes wide open and eyebrows high. 'I'm not saying anyone should give up western medicine, that'd be silly. But there must be more connection between science-based approaches and other approaches. How lonely does it feel in a doctor's waiting room or even in the appointment itself? How often do we know to go with our gut? Our bodies know ourselves better than anyone.'

'Well, that is really interesting. Thank you for telling me that.'

Clio reaches over and takes my hand. Hers is smooth and cool. Like a mother's hand.

'Lucy, I wanted you to know that even if your worst fear comes to pass – and in all likelihood it'll never happen – but even if it does, there are alternatives to your dad's experience. There are other protocols that can be followed, that have helped people, thousands if not millions of people, all over the world. Just because your local GP or even the oncologist doesn't know about it, doesn't mean it's not real. It is real. It happened to me. So please don't let this fear control you. You can live a life without fear.'

She squeezes my hand and I feel cared for. It's the loveliest feeling.

'Thank you so much. That means a lot to me. Thanks for sharing that with me, Clio.'

She pats my hand and leans back.

But I want to know more. 'So, can I ask you one more question?'

'Sure.'

'Is that how you got into wellness stuff? Or were you doing it before?'

'That's exactly how I got into it. I wasn't interested in anything to do with wellness before my cancer. I was a chartered surveyor by trade, for domestic houses. I hated my job. But beating cancer changed everything for me. I set up my new business, with only enough money for the next six months in my bank account and here I am today with the best annual earnings I've ever had, by a mile. I run this therapy strand of my business, plus I have a public speaking role too, where I'm asked to come and give inspirational speeches about my life and work. I travel and I get to work from home too, both of which I love to do. And I love how I can help people become their best selves. It's the best job in the world.'

141

'Wow . . . ' is all I manage to say. Clio sure is living the dream. And helping people too. I wish I could say the same. But instead, at my job, everybody acts like they can't stand the bloody sight of me. How nice it would be to have people who were grateful to you, instead of shouting at you just for doing your job. 'I wish I could say the same!'

Then Clio glances at her watch and says, 'I'm sorry, Lucy, but we've only got a few minutes left. Do you feel okay now?'

'I do, thanks so much. It's been amazing today. Harrowing! But amazing.'

I hate the fact these sessions feel so short. I want to talk with her more about her cancer treatment and everything she did to get well. It sounds incredible. I just need to know more. What an extraordinary woman.

'Good, good,' says Clio. 'I mean, the harrowing part might not feel good! But change is necessary and change is often painful. I hope you get something out of it. I have a feeling you will.'

'Definitely,' I reply. 'I'll be booking another session for next Friday, if that's okay?'

'Yes, of course. I'll look forward to it.'

We stand up and she's about to walk me to the door when she says, 'Ah, there's one more thing I meant to mention. I usually do tell my clients this once they've been a couple of times and want to come more regularly. I have an app – Clarity with Clio – that you can access if you wish. I designed it myself based on my own therapies. It's a kind of online journal where you can record your weekly thoughts after each session and the app will use AI to give you affirmations and advice.'

'That sounds great. How brilliant that you designed it yourself!'

This woman's talents are pretty impressive.

'Ah, thanks. It took years of research and investment but it was worth it. My clients find it so helpful. It's £10 a month for the first month as a bonus and thereafter £25 a month. Please think of it as an extension of these sessions. I check in on everyone's entries and the affirmations given and tweak when necessary. So you get a lot for your fee, I make sure of that.'

'Sign me up!' I say. I mean, it's not cheap but I really want to have it now she's explained it.

'Great. I'll send you the link tonight.'

Clio walks to my car and unexpectedly gives me a hug.

'You've been so brave today, Lucy. I'm so proud of the work you're doing here. And you should be proud of yourself too.'

With that, she walks back to the house. I sit in the car for a minute, a bit overwhelmed. I realise that this woman has rewritten the book of wellness for me and I'm hugely impressed by her. It makes me think about how many times my doctor – or a friend's doctor or even my dad's doctors – got things wrong or the medical system let them down and people suffered as a result. Everything Clio says makes perfect sense. Wow, she's inspirational. I did not expect to feel like this. Am I becoming a wellness junkie?! If I am, and if Clio is involved, then I don't care. Tara was absolutely right: it is life-changing. And I am totally here for it.

Chapter 13

The following morning, on Saturday, I'm in bed again with the newspapers, my usual routine. But this morning, I'm brooding. I'm worried. I'm thinking ahead to our staff conference at the end of March. Somehow, I've got to give the speech of my life. About wellness, something I know fuck all about, apart from the random few sessions I've attended. I need help, but who can help me with this? The only person I know who has a clue about wellness is Tara Harryman and obviously I'm not asking my rival for help, no way. I feel like I'll be bullshitting my way through it to dozens of people, including the old and new CEOs, both of which I need to impress madly to be in with a chance of netting this job. But what the hell can I do in that speech to engage them and the whole crowd? Cartwheels? Pole dancing?! Fuck, if only. I simply don't know what I'm going to do and it's making me anxious as hell.

I only feel better when Clio's link to the app pops up on my phone. Ooh! Let's have a go at this then. I download the

144

app. Once I'm in, I make an account, sign in and I have a little look around it. It has healthy recipes – oh good! I'll need those on my healthy eating plan I've just this morning decided to embark upon – and then a section where you have to write your entries after your session. The app gives you prompts of questions: *How useful was tonight's session? What did you learn about yourself? How will you put this into practice to help increase your wellbeing? What small change would you like to implement in your life this week?* I fill all that lot in, full of praise for the session which really did blow my mind. I press Enter and then the app gives me my advice, in three parts:

Try reaching out to your family. Maybe they're waiting for you to take the first step.

Wow, I'm pretty taken aback that the AI has come up with that. I mean, I know I put in info about my dad but truthfully it's what I've been thinking about for a while now, how to mend things with Mum and Shirl. Clio must've trained her AI well.

The next one is:

*Family issues can cause a lot of stress which will affect your sleep. Click **here** for the solution.*

Well, it's not wrong. My family does cause me to stress out plus my sleep is pretty rubbish, ever since the menopause. I click on the link and it takes me to Amazon to buy some lavender pillow spray for good sleeping. Okay, why not? Well, it is £18 . . . but its RRP is £26, so that's a bargain, isn't it? Yeah, fuck it. I click on Buy Now.

The last piece of advice is:

You might want to look into eating a broader diet of rainbow foods, do you agree?

Well, yeah, I suppose so. I mean, I must admit, I do eat quite a lot of beige i.e. far too many carbs, I'm guessing. I haven't had breakfast yet, so when I go downstairs, I spot my usual Saturday treats of croissants on the side and I realise they're beige too. I suddenly really, really don't want to eat them. So I open the fridge door and stare inside, hoping the right answer will present itself. I notice the blueberries and raspberries I usually pick up to have with the croissants. They're rainbow foods for sure, I mean, what other foods are blue? Are there any? And everything red seems to be good for you. Then I think about what I can put with them. In the end, I prepare a bowl of no-added-sugar granola, yoghurt with a spoon of almond butter stirred in, plus the fresh berries. The granola in my cupboard has been there for about nine months, since my last attempt at living more healthily lasted about three days. I always have the other stuff in, as I like adding yoghurt to takeaway curries if they're too spicy plus I love almond butter spread thickly on white toast (more beigeness, but surely nut butter is pretty damn good for you. Healthy fats, and all that?). I feel virtuous after that breakfast. I wonder how long this attempt at healthy eating will last. Until the moment I miss the salty scent of frying bacon, most likely.

I don't have any plans for today. I know I could use the time to call my family in New Zealand. But I'll have to wait till this evening for that, due to the time difference. And I'm not even sure I want to. It's always so draining. So I decide to go and see another family member instead. I haven't visited this person for a while, which has been wracking me with guilt, so I pop by the local florist on the way and buy a nice couple of pots of hyacinth bulbs, just starting to push through the soil into the world. Everyone likes hyacinths. I head north of town to a place called Southborough and park up. I walk down the path, flanked by bare winter trees. There's the odd bulb pushing through the soil here too. Spring can't be too far away then. It's not long before I reach my destination. My father's grave.

Albert Cooper
Beloved father
Devoted husband

Mum chose that for his grave. It's so bland. Doesn't tell you anything about him. I wish it'd said something real about him, something that could tell him apart from every other damn grave in the lot.

Addicted to custard creams
Always chose the boot in Monopoly

I mean, who else chooses the boot in Monopoly?! I read on a Facebook post recently that it was retired as a piece a few years back, along with the thimble and wheelbarrow. Apparently they were replaced with a penguin, a rubber ducky and a T-Rex.

Modern life is fucking stupid.

I bend down to clear some dead leaves from his grave and then pop the hyacinth pots in front of the stone.

'There you go, you old codger,' I say.

And as soon as I've said that, I'm in tears, just like last night. Seeing him again in Clio's session made him real for me once more, whereas the hard and hollow truth is that he's here, a collection of bones, beneath this scrubby grass, in this dank earth.

I don't want to cry in front of him. I'm supposed to be

cheering him up, aren't I? I hold back the tears. I can do that for him, at least.

'Well, then, me old matey,' I begin, wiping my eyes. 'It's me. Sorry I haven't been for a while. It's been a miserable winter, as I'm sure you're aware. I bet you hear all sorts of weather sweeping above you while you're cosy below. Lots of rain and fog. Not that cold. That's global warming for you. But just . . . bleak. That's the word for it, like "In the Bleak Midwinter", your favourite Christmas carol. We could've put that on your gravestone too.'

I ought to tell him about Mum's heart attack, or not heart attack. I know I should tell him how Shirl is and her kids. But I don't want to admit that I don't keep up with them enough and I don't want to think about them very often. I know he'd bring up the time when he was near the end but still compos mentis and he told me I should go with them to New Zealand, which he knew Shirl and her husband had wanted to do for years. Start a new life. He knew my marriage was on the skids and he wanted me to escape. But then, who would be here to talk to him if I'd buggered off too, eh? Nobody, that's who. So, here I am. Better late than never.

'But look, Dad, I am sorry I've not been for a while, since Christmas Day. Work has been hectic, as usual. I know you always said I worked too hard. You're not wrong. I've only got worse with that since we lost you. I don't know, Dad . . . I just feel like it's my life, my work. And I was holding out, all these years, for that COO post. And do you know what, Dad? Those fuckers might take it away from me, at the very last hurdle. I won't bore you with the details but this new woman at work might get it instead of me. I can't believe it, after all my years of service. But look, Dad, I'm not going to let those bastards beat me. I'm a fighter, like you always said about me. Determined, driven. I will reach the pinnacle of my career, I'm sure of that. Just need to ace this wellness stuff, then I'm home free.'

I explain wellness to him because he won't have heard of it. I don't even know if we used that word seven years ago. Maybe before that it was one of those words like couth or ruth that doesn't ever get used without its negative bit, uncouth or ruthless. Maybe wellness as the opposite of illness is a new thing. Either way, Dad would never understand this obsession we all have now with optimising our bodies and minds. He'd think it was a load of old crap.

'Maybe you're right, Dad. And that's what I thought at first. A load of bollocks sold by grifters. But I've met this extraordinary woman called Clio. She had cancer, like you, Dad. And she had surgery but then she refused chemo. She went into remission, by ignoring doctors and doing her own thing with nutrition. Amazing, really. I wish we'd known about your cancer sooner and knew about Clio's methods. Maybe we could've . . . had you around . . . a bit longer . . .'

I'm going to start sobbing if I'm not careful. I pull myself together and carry on.

'Truth is, Dad, I need some wellness in my life. I've been living mired in unhealthy habits for too long. I need to start a new way of living, I think. And don't worry – I'll still have a custard cream every now and again. I've not gone completely soft. But this wellness stuff isn't all as daft as it sounds. You just have to sift out the scammers from the real deal. That's what I'm doing, Dad. Trying to make a better version of myself. I hope you'd be proud of me. I'm evolving. And with Clio's help, I don't feel so alone on that journey.'

The wind on this cold, early February day whips up all of a sudden and blows a bunch of dead leaves across his grave again.

'If that's you controlling the weather to make a point, then you can stop that. I know we used to take the piss out of people who talked about going on spiritual journeys – I remember us laughing at celebrities who joined cults, like Tom Cruise and Scientology. You always said about him that he was dead behind the eyes. But look, that's not me, you know that. I'm smarter than that. I'm not buying into some ridiculous wellness cult. I'm still me, Dad. Still the same foul-mouthed bitchy cynic you loved. Just trying something new. It's about time for it. It's all good. Plus it's going to help me nail this job, Dad. Just you watch me. By the staff conference – with Clio's help – I'll be the foremost expert on wellness and I'll work out a way to impress the old CEO and the new one so much, that Tara won't stand a bloody chance. All right, yeah, the staff will be sick of listening to me. They can't stand me, most of them. But somehow, I will make them sit up and listen. How are you going to do that, I hear you say? Well, Dad, I don't know how I'll do it yet exactly, but . . .'

I'm struggling because I really don't bloody know. My anxiety from this morning comes back. How am I going to make a splash at this damn thing? But then I stop. I've just had a thought. I know I am going to do a speech about wellness. But then I realise that the whole thing would be tons better if I had another keynote speaker on wellness to really make our staff sit up and listen. Someone who's inspirational . . . compelling . . . experienced . . . magnetic – and I'm not talking about shoving magnets up your arse.

'Dad, you're brilliant! That's it! I'll ask Clio to be our

keynote speaker! Didn't she say she was a public speaker? She did! And the CEOs will love it! Derek always did have a weakness for strong women, so I know he'll think Clio is fabulous. I can just see her now, talking about her wellness journey, beating cancer, for fuck's sake! That's so inspirational, the crowd will love it. Thanks, Dad. Love you so much, you clever bastard, you!'

Dad says nothing, obviously. But I know he'd be grinning from ear to ear if he were by my side.

Give 'em hell, he'd say.

Oh I will, Dad . . . That'll be one in the eye for perfect Tara and her perfect life, hashtag wellness warrior – oh fuck off! I'll have Clarity with Clio on my side. If Derek agrees to her speaker's fee . . . and if Clio says yes, that is . . .

Monday morning comes and I'm beating down Derek's office door first thing, but he's not in yet. I've already had a look at Clio's website. Turns out her name is Clio Kenton and she has a separate tab on her site for inspirational talks and her fee for an hour's speech including Q&A is . . . £700. I mean, that's quite a bit of money . . . but not too bad considering some people's fees. But our budget for the conference, including the venue and refreshments, is pretty fixed, so I need to check that Derek's happy to okay it.

'Eager beaver this morning, Lucia,' says Derek as he trundles along to his office, a half-hour late as I'm loitering around chatting with Sharon, awaiting his tardy arrival.

'Something rather urgent to discuss with you,' I say and he looks momentarily worried. 'No cause for concern. A rather great idea of mine I want to run past you.'

'Sure, fire away,' says Derek as I follow him into his office

151

and he shuts the door. We sit, him behind his vast desk and me opposite him.

'Regarding the staff conference at the end of next month. I've noticed a definite downturn in staff morale and behaviour in the past few months. And since news of the new CEO there's been even more concern, with rumours about redundancies abounding, even though we have no firm updates on that as yet. So, I really feel that this year's conference has some heavy lifting to do in terms of morale and engendering optimism and community spirit going forward at Beane & Co.'

'Agreed! They're like a bunch of unruly sailors out there. If we're not careful, there'll be demands for us to walk the plank soon! This lot needs whipping into shape.'

Not exactly the metaphor I'd go for, but at least he's agreeing with me.

'So, with that in mind, I'd like to make a proposal. I will of course be doing my own speech on wellness, as agreed. However, I'd like to request in addition to this a keynote speaker from outside the organisation, someone inspirational, someone to bring back a sense of optimism to our staff, someone who can invigorate them and make them see that there are ways they can improve their own lives, that we at Beane & Co can work in tandem with that in their work lives too.'

'Sounds marvellous. Who is it?'

'Her name is Clio Kenton and she runs her own wellness business, built from scratch after her cancer diagnosis.'

'Cancer?' says Derek. He looks concerned. Maybe he's worried it sounds a bit depressing.

'Clio beat cancer with the help of her own wellness methods and now does inspirational speeches all about it. So no, it's not depressing at all. Her story is truly inspiring and she herself has a wonderful way about her. A truly impressive person who's been in the depths and come back fighting. I think it's just the kind of lift our staff need.'

'Well, that sounds . . . interesting.' He's looking into the middle distance, considering something.

'I think it will be very interesting, Derek.'

'This woman, Clio . . . ?'

'Kenton.'

'Yes. She cured her own cancer, you say?'

'Well, I don't know the exact details, except that she had surgery and then refused the follow-up treatment and turned to her own methods instead. Mostly to do with nutrition, I think.'

'Nutrition,' he repeats.

'Yes . . . so, shall we book Clio Kenton as our speaker, if you think it sounds like a good idea?'

'Yes, absolutely. And I trust your judgement, Lucia, you know that. Cost?'

I pause briefly before I throw the number at him. '£700.'

Derek replies, 'Well, it's not cheap. But I've heard worse, far worse. And if you're telling me you can vouch for this person . . . is that the case?'

'Yes, absolutely.'

'Then, I say yes to that, Lucia. Let's bring her in. We will present a united front of strong women at work. I'm sure you know me well enough after all these years to say how much I value strong women in the workplace, Lucia, yourself included.'

I do know him far too well and also know his penchant for strong women in the workplace is almost a kind of fetish.

'Of course.'

'I mean, just look at you and Tara. It's marvellous to see you two head-to-head for the top post under the new CEO. I can't wait to see how that one turns out! Nick Bridges will have the choice of a lifetime on his hands between you two! Tara has already made so many positive changes to the business, saving us money left, right and centre, as well as introducing legal safeguards for which we were rather behind the times. You'll have to limber up to beat Tara in this battle, eh? I can see getting a smashing new keynote speaker for the conference strengthens your case on that score. Very good. Very nicely done, Lucia!'

Urgh. To hear Derek banging on about Tara and all her virtues makes me nauseous. Yes, she has introduced some money-saving tips to the business but her new legal safeguards have cost us a load of money too, which Derek doesn't seem to understand. Plus most of the things she's implemented have caused a bunch of extra work for the directors, including me, so we're all pissed off about that. I've heard the odd middle manager mention her name in the corridor with a touch of venom about the additional workload she's piled up for them. Anyway, the important thing is, Derek has said yes.

'Thanks, Derek. Much appreciated. I do believe we're going to have the best staff conference ever this year.'

'I do hope so, considering it'll be my last! I really want to go out with a bang. I'm relying on you to ensure that happens, Lucia!'

I stand up to go, reassuring him that I'm one hundred per cent certain it will, when the door opens and Sharon shows someone in . . . well, well, well. If it isn't my mud-fight opponent Tara Harryman. Always showing up everywhere and never welcome, like dog shit.

'Lucy, Derek,' says Tara, with the fakest of fake smiles.

'Your 9.45,' says Sharon to Derek, yet eyeing me, because I didn't make an appointment, which is why she's shown Tara in without even knocking as Sharon is annoyed with me for messing up her schedule.

'I'll let you get on, Derek,' I say.

'Tara!' cries Derek as if she's the second coming, which she probably thinks she is. 'Exciting news from Lucia. Tell her!'

He's directing me and Tara is looking at me, expectantly, suspiciously. She knows anything that benefits me probably won't do the same for her.

'I'm going to ask Clio Kenton to be our keynote speaker for the staff conference,' I say smugly, though well aware that Clio hasn't said yes yet.

Tara doesn't miss a beat and goes straight in with, 'If she has the time for it. And you have left it rather last minute, Lucy. She's a highly sought-after inspirational speaker, you know.'

Derek pipes up, 'Oh, you know this venerable lady as well, do you, Tara?'

'Yes, Clio is part of the wellness bootcamp that Lucy and I have undertaken. I've continued to see her beyond the January Rejuvenate course because . . . well, she's just brilliant.'

I didn't know Tara was having extra sessions with Clio too. This somehow annoys me immeasurably. I wanted to feel like Clio was my special discovery. But then, I remember, it was by stalking Tara's socials that I found out about the bootcamp in the first place, which led me to Clio. And I can see by the look on her face that Tara's annoyed with me too.

It's clear that she feels the same way about Clio's sessions as I do. Well, good, because now Tara will be even more annoyed by me getting Clio in. God, I hope Clio says yes, after all this, because if she says no, I'll be the loser. Damn it.

'Marvellous,' says Derek. 'Hop to it then, Lucia.'

Lucia . . . the last time that bloody man calls me Lucia before he sashays off to the great golden golf course of the retired will be the happiest moment of my life.

I go straight to my desk and craft an email to Clio making the offer of the speech with all the requisite details. Within an hour, I see a reply pop up:

It would be my pleasure, Lucy. I would love to accept your invitation to speak at your staff conference on 28th March. We can discuss more on Friday – do come ten minutes early so we have a bit of extra time. See you then.

Fuck yeah!!

Chapter 14

Friday comes and I'm in like Flint, arriving fifteen minutes early. I have to make way for another car coming out of Clio's drive before I can go in. I squint at it as it passes, to see if it's Tara but I can't tell; it's a large Mercedes and I'm pretty sure Tara has a Mazda MX-5, as a new one has started parking in our work car park in the last few weeks. I pull up and find Clio at the door, awaiting me.

Inside, we have a quick chat about the staff conference.

I say to Clio, 'I'm so sorry it's a bit last minute, I mean, six weeks is not much notice.'

'Not at all. It was a lovely surprise. I have another client who works at that company, funnily enough. I can't say who due to confidentiality, of course.'

Urgh. Of course I know who she means. And I'd imagine Clio shouldn't have even said that, should she, if she wants to be confidential? But anyway, it doesn't matter, as I know who it is. It is my nemesis.

'Ah, I know. Tara Harryman. She was the one who told

157

me about the bootcamp in the first place.' Slight white lie . . .

'Oh, good. I'm glad you know each other. It'll be a pleasure to see you both at the staff conference. Two extraordinary women owning the workplace. I'm proud to be working with both you and Tara.'

Well, that would be a lovely compliment if Tara's damn name wasn't uttered in the same sentence. Anyway, we talk a bit more about what kind of things she could speak about and I tell her I really don't mind, as long as it's something inspirational to give our staff a kick up the arses.

'They really are the most recalcitrant bunch,' I add. 'Makes my job extremely vexing. I really appreciate your input at the conference.'

'I can see you're really struggling with your feelings about work at the moment. In tonight's session, we can think about that, yet also there are lots of issues to work through concerning your father. I think it might also be worth considering the rest of your family too and how things have been with them since his passing, seeing whether there could be some healing there.'

'Urgh,' I utter involuntarily. 'My family isn't . . . easy. Mum and my sister Shirl and her family moved to New Zealand a year after Dad's death. I never really got on with either of them, especially Mum. Dad was my rock. Shirl and Mum were a pair, still are. They said I should come to New Zealand with them but I didn't. I didn't want to.'

'That's fascinating. There's certainly a lot there to unpick. Especially concerning your relationship with your mother, I'd say.'

'Well, I'd rather not, to be honest! I know how I feel about all that and none of it is good.'

'I'm sorry to hear that,' says Clio, her face full of sympathy. 'I'm aware of time again so shall we get going? I want you to have as much time as possible in your visions tonight.'

We go through the usual routine except this time I harbour a slight apprehension at what might be behind that door down the corridor, because the first one was a whole other life entirely, whereas the second was my own life. What will it be this time?

I open the door and I'm coming out of a bathroom onto a dim carpeted landing of a small house, the sound of a toilet filling up behind me. The carpet is brown and looking up I see the walls are brown too. I'm definitely in the twentieth century, and when I peer down the stairs, I can see a hall table near the front door with a curly-wired rotary telephone placed on it, joined to the wall. Maybe it's the seventies, considering the chocolate colour scheme. I peek back into the bathroom and see the toilet, bath and sink are all avocado green. Yes, definitely the 1970s or early 80s. I look down at myself and see I'm wearing a yellow cotton summer frock, sleeveless, with a print of little bunches of red cherries dotted about on the skirt. I'm slim and quite short. I raise my hand and touch my hair. It's pinned back in some kind of chignon, neat and held in place by sticky lacquered layers of hairspray. From the next room beside the bathroom comes a sound. Like gurgling. Then a little cry. It's a baby. I freeze. I know in my heart that I cannot cope with that baby waking up right now. It's the first break I've had all day and I'm exhausted. My three-year-old daughter has just gone down for a nap too in her bedroom and the last thing I need is the baby waking her up as well. I just need ten damn minutes to myself. I never get any bloody time to myself!

Wow, this desperation has filled me with anxiety, yet as the baby sounds abate and silence returns, pure relief sweeps over me. I tiptoe downstairs as quietly as possible and go into the kitchen. It's a warm spring day, I can see it through the kitchen window into the garden. There's a square of lawn, perfectly mown, and beds surrounding it with a variety of perennial shrubs in, including my pale peach tea roses. There are some raised beds by the patio with seedlings ready to grow into crops of vegetables. My garden is my pride and joy. If I wasn't a housewife and mother, I know that I'd want to be a gardener, or more specifically, run my own plant nursery. I started growing seeds when I was a little girl, back in the late forties, after the war. My grandfather helped me. He loved his garden. It was L-shaped and had a little greenhouse where he grew cucumbers that hung down on stalks and bunches of grapes that lined the roof inside the hothouse. I'd go and help him at weekends, especially after Sunday school as his house was down the road from my father's church.

I put the kettle on and make myself a cup of Mellow Bird's coffee, with a spoonful of Coffeemate creamer, as well as a dash of milk. I would love a spoon of sugar but I mustn't. I don't want to get fat. My father always made it clear to me that the worst of the seven sins was gluttony. And a fat woman was a failed woman. That's what he said to me, that's what he preached. And he did talk to us like that, my father. As if he was up in his pulpit. I feel my hips and stomach. I know I've put on weight since I had the baby – not too much – but I must stick to my diet now. Half a grapefruit for breakfast, no sugar. Boiled egg, slice of ham and carrot sticks for lunch. Then whatever it is I'm making my husband for dinner, I'll have the same, but about half the portion. He needs to eat a big dinner as he works so hard. I work hard too. But nobody sees it that way. Housework isn't real work, is it?

I must admit, I have stood on the front doorstep, the baby on one arm, the little one holding on to my skirts as we wave their daddy goodbye for the day and I've watched his Austin Princess recede down the close and disappear around the corner – and I am so bloody envious of him, I could scream. I want him to stay here and deal with all this, with the housework and the screaming, demanding kiddies hanging on me all day and all night. I want to waltz off to an office to push paper around. It's not fair. Why do women get all the horrid jobs? Why do I feel dead inside when I'm at home, much of the time? Why is the only time I truly feel alive when I'm pruning the roses in the garden, or pulling up weeds, or slotting bedding plants into warm soil, or sowing seeds for the carrots and peas the children will eat raw from the ground, after a little wash under the garden hose? Why couldn't I have gone to university and studied botany, as I always wanted to?

Because my father insisted that I was stupid, that's why. That I was good for nothing but a secretary's job, if that. So I learnt to type. And I worked at my husband-to-be's office. And I married him. Because he was nice enough and a good match and because it was what everyone expected of me. And then the babies came and I was stuck forever, in this life that I never wanted.

I sigh a long drawn-out sigh and take a sip of my coffee. It tastes so much better with sugar. But needs must. I was a fat little thing as a girl and my father never let me forget it. Oh, I do hope neither of my daughters turn out fat or I'll just want to die. I can't cope with that. I can't let them be the failure that I was. Then, I hear the one sound I can't bear to hear. The baby has woken up. And she's screaming. Why on earth do babies need to scream? They have their every need taken care of every second of every day and night. What do they have to scream about? I'm the one who needs to have a good long scream. I have been miscast in the role of mother. I love my daughters, of course I do. I'd die for them, in a heartbeat, without a second thought. But that doesn't take away the feeling that I was destined to be the guardian not to two human girls, but instead to a greenhouse full of seedlings, a row of greenhouses in my specialist plant nursery, focusing on my favourites: alpines and ferns. Grandpa taught me all about them. I knew all the Latin names. That feels like lost knowledge now, ancient knowledge, gone in the mists of time, just as Grandpa is long gone. I feel close to him when I'm in my garden. My happy place. My tiny domestic homage to the plant nursery I know deep down I should be running. That's where I know I should be, not here, standing in my kitchen drinking tasteless coffee and listening to that infant screaming about nothing upstairs. And now my three-year-old is screaming for me too. She's crying. She's upset the baby has woken her up. She wants her mummy. I just want to run away and never come back. I'd never do that, of course, but it doesn't stop me wanting it.

'I'm coming!' I shout up the stairs, as nicely as I can, as brightly as I can, putting on the pretence of motherhood like I put on a raincoat for a storm. I pour my coffee down the drain, as I didn't want it anyway, not without lovely sugar. Back I go upstairs, with a feeling of dread in the pit of my stomach, as I call out, 'It's all right, Lucy. Mummy's coming. Let's go and see your sister, baby Shirley. See if we can make her smile.'

Chapter 15

Everything goes black then and I'm instantaneously back in the corridor. I want to go back to that house. I try the door and it's locked.

'Why is it locked?' I cry to Clio.

'There will be a reason,' is Clio's mysterious reply.

I open my eyes. I'm back in the therapy room. I'm not crying, I'm not emotional. I'm just blown away by what I just saw and experienced.

'So,' says Clio. 'Was that your mother?'

'Yes!' I say. 'As a young woman. I must've been three and Shirl was a baby. So . . . 1975. Mum would've been thirty-three. I can't believe it! It was . . . incredible. To hear her thoughts, her hopes and dreams. My God, I had no idea.'

'Was all of that news to you?'

I think hard about this.

'Well, no, now I come to think of it. Since I'm not sure that I really believe in past-life regression, I'd have to say that this jump into my mum's past was built on my own memories of her. Not when I was three, but the things she's said to me since and the comments she's made about her own life.'

'What kind of thing?'

'Well, about how she always wanted to be a horticulturalist. How her father – a pretty strict and unpleasant vicar, by all accounts – I never knew him as he died when I was very young, can't remember what year – anyway, her father was against it. She did love her garden and spent as much time in it as she could. She loved her grandpa too and mentioned him often. She told me once she wished I'd met him, as he was such a kind, sweet man with "infinite patience", she said. She was a housewife for years when we were little and we loved it, of course, because she was always there to pick us up from school and come to our little plays or recorder concerts or whatever. She was always just . . . there. And when we were older and we didn't need her so much, she looked a bit lost. She got a job for a while at the local corner shop and it was weird to go in and see your own mother behind the counter. Dad worked in insurance, just as I do now, following in his footsteps. He used to tell her she didn't need to work but I got the impression she needed it. When we left home, before Shirl had her babies quite a bit later towards the end of her thirties, Mum volunteered in a community garden before Dad got sick. She was happier then, those few years. God, it kills me to think of her so unhappy when we were little.'

Clio asks, 'Were you aware of it then?'

'No, not really. She was a good mum. Critical, though, and quite judgemental. Especially about the fat thing. It was always an issue in our house – not with Dad, he didn't give a stuff about it and was pretty chunky himself before he got ill. But Mum was always going on about food and calories and weighing herself. I once went snooping in her cupboard for something and found a piece of graph paper Blu-tacked to the inside of the door, with a weight loss chart on it but the line kept going up and I thought how depressing it must be to see that every morning, despite your best efforts. She never ate much, not in front of us anyway. I do remember seeing a bag of toffees in her bedside drawer and stealing one. I was terrible for rooting around in her stuff. I took money from her purse too. God, what an awful thing to do! What a little shit I was. But then I suppose I was acting out to get her attention, because her attention was always – always – on Shirley. I always found my mum a bit removed from me. She and Shirl got on like a house on fire. They just seemed to have a secret body language that I didn't understand. One would set the other off laughing and I'd be standing there saying "what?" and smiling, trying to be in on the joke but they'd never explain it to me. There was a lot I didn't tell my mum, stuff that happened at school or with boyfriends and whatever, because I knew she'd say "I told you so" and I couldn't bear hearing that from her. She always took such glee in it, as if she wanted the bad thing to happen just so she could be smug about it. But during our teens and beyond, once we were old enough to understand a bit more, I do remember her saying that when we were babies was the hardest period of her life. I guess once Shirl got older and they bonded so deeply, she was happier maybe, not so alone. She certainly didn't get any comfort from me.'

'You're very hard on yourself,' says Clio, leaning forward, crossed arms on her knees.

'Not really,' I say, staring past her at all the house plants on her window ledge, thinking of the time Mum told me about aeoniums and how to look after them. I've had them ever since in my house. 'She just likes Shirley more than me. But I had my dad, thank God.'

There's a pregnant pause then.

Clio says, 'It sounds to me as if she found motherhood very hard. Many women do. It's one of the last taboos, I think. We're taught that women are supposed to find parenthood easy, as a natural thing, mothering instinct and all that. I never had it. Never wanted children.'

'Me neither!'

'And we've had to bear the weight of other people's expectations with that too, that we're somehow lacking because of it.'

'Wait a minute . . . ' I sit up then, as something occurs to me, shuffling to get myself comfy sitting up on the chaise longue. 'Maybe Mum never really wanted kids either. I remember her telling me one day that it was just the done thing in the late sixties. Respectable women became wives and then mothers. Sounds like she didn't want either of those things. It was just what was expected of her. Honestly, the thought now of having teenagers at home and a husband fills me with horror. I chose to avoid all that. But Mum didn't even have that choice. I remember when I was doing my A levels and applying to uni and didn't really know what I wanted to do – archaeologist in the *Indiana Jones* vein or an expert on the *Antiques Roadshow* – she told me that whatever I decided, I could always change my mind later. But that the only irreversible decision was having a child.'

'Very true,' says Clio. 'When was the last time you spoke to your mother?'

I feel assaulted by guilt.

'Too long ago.'

Clio doesn't say anything but the air is heavy with the answer to this. But actually, I realise I want to speak to my mum. For the first time in ages, I feel curious to speak to her.

'Please don't feel guilty for that,' says Clio, smiling, making me feel less of a terrible daughter. 'Relationships with mothers and daughters are complex things. I left home myself at sixteen to escape my mother.'

'Really?'

Clio nods and sighs. It looks like she doesn't want to talk about it, but she carries on. 'Our relationship was pretty toxic. I left and never looked back. I had one sister, like you, but she was very close to my parents and I was always the odd one out. I walked out at sixteen and cut my family out of my life completely. Never saw any of them again. I'm not recommending that for everyone, of course. But it worked for me. I had to struggle to make it through life after that. I actually am glad for that struggle now. It made me a much stronger person. I had to work at several jobs at once from sixteen onwards. I learnt the value of a work ethic. Now I want to pay that forward to other women, to earn just enough for my own life to live how I need to and the rest all goes back into research for my work. Leaving my mother was the making of me. But I don't sense that for you, Lucy.'

'Please, call me Lu,' I say. Clio knows so much about me now, I feel like she should call me by the name I consider to be the real me.

'Okay, thank you, Lu. Yes, so for you, I think your relationship with your mother sounds eminently salvageable. And with your sister too. Would you agree? Tell me about how your vision today might help with that.'

167

'I would, actually. Being in mum's shoes . . . it's been a gift to me, it really has. I feel like I had a tiny window into her existence anyway, that desperation I felt, to be alone with my own thoughts and inclinations. That sinking feeling when the kids woke up. Wow. I really recognised that deep sense of frustration and exhaustion that she felt at that moment. Not with kids, but with the people I have to manage at work, who – believe me – act like children a lot of the time. I feel like their work mother much of the time too. But at least I can walk away from it each evening at five-thirty. Mum couldn't do that with her kids. Thank you, Clio. I can't tell you how grateful I am to you for this.'

Clio then gestures towards me. 'None of this was me. All of it came from you. You have travelled to these places and chosen to go through that door. I was just the facilitator.'

'Well, you're a shit-hot facilitator then!'

We both laugh. Then Clio shifts forward in her seat and looks intently at me.

'Listen, Lu, we're nearly out of time. But I have something I'd like to ask you. An invitation, if you will.'

Sounds dead intriguing. 'Oh yeah?'

'Yes, I'm holding a wellness retreat next weekend, taking place at Roseland Hall in the countryside near here. Some of my other clients will be there – I only invite those clients who I feel will get the most out of it, as numbers are tight and I can't invite everyone. I only usually invite clients of mine that I've had for years, but I'm making an exception for you because you really have proven to me that this process has been incredibly useful for you in highlighting your current issues and the way you've taken to it is like a fish to the ocean. I've been tremendously impressed by your responses.

I think this wellness retreat could be marvellous for you and I'd welcome your input during our group sessions there. Only if you're interested, of course.'

A few weeks ago, if someone told me I'd be nigh on falling off a chaise longue with keenness to go on a wellness retreat weekend with someone called Clio – I'd have told them to fuck off. But it's true! And of course I'm interested!

'Oh wow, yes please! I'd love to come.'

'Are you sure you can make it? I know how hard you work.'

'Oh, I can definitely make it. And it'll be a really useful experience for the wellness speech I'm going to make at the staff conference. Thank you so much for inviting me!'

'You're welcome. There is quite a substantial cost, of course, as it's two nights' accommodation and all meals included. Also included in the price are my own group sessions. I'll send you the link later and you can see the prices and decide accordingly.'

I think of my savings squirrelled away for a rainy day. And I think of how much I might pay for a repair to my car or the cost of all the takeaways I've had in a year, plus delivery charges for random food late at night while I'm working. All money spent on things that won't change my life, but I know that this will. Whatever the cost of this retreat, I will be going.

Clio and I say our goodbyes as the session has come to its end. Back home after the session, I immediately go on my phone and see if she's sent the link yet, but no luck so far. I'm sure she'll do it soon. A wellness retreat with Clio! How thrilling!

I cook myself a stir fry with veg and chicken I got from the Co-op yesterday, as well as some very old Super Noodles in my cupboard and a packet of black bean sauce that's also a bit ancient. It tastes really good, actually and must be better for you than getting it from a takeaway. Then, later in the evening, it occurs to me, it's just the right time for a call to New Zealand, as it's 11am Saturday there and everybody should be off work and school. I could message Shirl and ask her to set up a video call some time with Mum and me and her and Noah and Ned, and also Shirl's husband, Ray. I'm not a big fan of video calls but, having said that, it would actually be so nice to see them all, see those smiling faces who look a bit like mine, and remember that I do have a family after all. I'm not, in fact, an orphan, even if I feel like one much of the time. But I feel if I message Shirl first, she'll find a reason to put it off.

So I don't give Shirley a chance to micro-manage and instead just tap on WhatsApp videocall and wait and see what happens next.

It rings for a while, a long time. Doesn't look like Shirl is going to answer it. I mean, I would normally never take an unsolicited video call. In fact, I'd stare at it in horror and say, *Who the fuck thinks it's appropriate to force themselves into my space with their face?* But this time, it's me doing the forcing and honestly, I don't care. I really want to speak to Mum.

Finally, Shirley answers.

I'm assaulted with an extreme close-up of Shirley's chin. She then pulls out and squints at the phone screen. Then she sees me, grinning like a maniac. As much as she annoys me, it's actually really nice to see my sister's old face. She's kept the colour from her youth, the dark brown hair we both inherited from our dad. Seeing how dark it is with the line of grey roots starting to show, it makes me glad that I've embraced the grey. Shirl must not be ready for that yet. I wish I could explain to her how liberating it is to get rid of the box dye and just be yourself. But she'd probably accuse me of interfering in her life. She is usually accusing me of something or other. Our relationship seems to have turned to vinegar as the years have gone by, rather than developing into a fine wine. But being in that vision earlier tonight makes me feel protective of little baby Shirley, while I was napping in my room. And here is that little sister, all grown up and laden with world weariness. She was just a screaming ball of neediness once with a shitty nappy. As were we all.

'Shirl!' I say and honestly, my eyes are pricked with tears.

'What's the matter? What's happened?'

She looks worried, as usual. Her whole life seems to be a litany of worries.

'Nothing's happened! I just wanted to see your face. And Mum's.'

'Stop being weird. Are you drunk? I suppose it is Friday night. How many bottles of red have you had?'

'None!' I cry, proud of myself as I actually forwent a glass or two tonight. I just didn't fancy it. 'How are you, Shirl?'

'Very, very busy, if you must know,' she says, holding the phone at an odd angle and looking past it into something that's going on beyond the camera.

'Shirl, hold your camera up as all I can see is right up your nostrils.'

She tuts and looks into the phone again. 'Look, it's lousy timing. We're having a barbecue and Ray's on the meat and the kids are not helping and Mum's hungry.'

'Can I see the kids?'

171

Shirley rolls her eyes. I hate it when she does that, like I'm the naughty child despite being three years older than her.

'Noah. Ned.' She shouts sharply, like she's summoning a pair of spaniels. Nobody comes and Shirley doesn't explain what's going on.

Maybe this whole spontaneous call thing was a bad idea.

'It's okay, Shirl, if they don't want to come,' I say loudly, but Shirl doesn't seem to hear me. Then the phone screen goes haywire as it's grabbed by someone and the next face I see is my fourteen-year-old nephew Noah. My God, I haven't seen him except in photos since last year and he's so different, it's shocking how fast they grow.

'Auntie L,' he says, face completely straight, except for a slight curve at the corner of his mouth.

'Nephew N,' I say and grin at him. He laughs then.

'Like all the memes?'

He sends them to me erratically on Insta and each and every one, though they must seem as inconsequential as a breadcrumb to him, are vastly enjoyed and appreciated by me.

'Bloody love them.'

He smiles briefly then says, 'Good. There's Ned, look. Being a twat.'

I hear Shirley's voice crying out in protest at Noah swearing, which he ignores, then deftly switches screen so I can see outward from Shirley's phone. I see a brief tableau of a family barbecue, a swathe of bright green grass, some exotic-looking plants with spears of leaves and flower spikes forcing their way upwards into the blue air, the sun beating down, Ray with tongs and apron, Ned on a vast expanse of decking – twelve years old and yet looking taller than me now – trying to do tricks on his skateboard. My heart aches to see them, my sweet nephews, doing their things, living their lives, so bloody far away. They were eight and six when they left and they used to hold my hand to cross the road and Ned still sat on my lap and asked me to read *The Hungry Caterpillar* to him, because I kept it from my childhood and would get it off the shelf for him over and over again. I used to tell them every time the hungry caterpillar went to his local restaurant on a buffet day they wouldn't let him in, because he'd scoff the whole damn buffet and there wouldn't be anything left for anyone else. Ned thought that was the height of wit. He used to fall off the sofa laughing. God, I miss them.

Then, Noah shifts the camera to briefly reveal my mother, seated in the shade of a parasol, at the edge of the decking, near the kitchen door. She's watching Ned on his skateboard too.

Noah must've lost interest as the phone goes straight back to Shirl and I see her worried face again.

'Can I speak to Mum?' I ask Shirl.

'No, she's upstairs, napping.'

'No, she isn't. She's on the decking. I just saw her!'

Shirley's face registers her clumsy lie and she shakes her head saying, 'She's about to go for a nap.'

'Just a quick hello, please?'

Why the hell do I need to beg my sister to speak to my own mother? It's ridiculous.

Shirley doesn't answer but the phone starts jogging up and down as she marches over there. She shoves the phone in Mum's face and says loudly, 'It's Lucy.'

Suddenly, I am presented with a close-up view of my

mother's old, wrinkled, heavily confused face. She doesn't know where to look. She doesn't know what's happening. She looks so much older than the last time I saw her. It's a shock to see her like that. She looks like a different person altogether.

'Mum!' I call out, hoping the sound of my voice will help to ground her.

'Lu-Lu?' she says, in a fragile way.

Oh, that's what my dad used to call me. Nobody has said that name in years.

'Yes,' I call out. 'It's Lu-Lu, Mum. Look at the phone. I'm here in the phone.'

Mum gazes downwards vaguely. She finally sees my face and hers changes. It's like the sun has come out.

'Lu-Lu,' she says and I can see her eyes are glinting in the strong New Zealand midday sunlight, glistening with tears.

'Hello, Mum,' I say and Christ, I'm crying too. How could I have left it so long? Yes, she's a bloody difficult woman, she always has been. But that's not much of an excuse.

'Hello, love,' she says, gently. I wish she'd spoken to me like that throughout my whole childhood. She so rarely did.

'How are you, Mum?'

Her pale blue eyes cloud a moment. 'I'm not always myself,' she says, haltingly.

'Sorry to hear that, Mum.'

Then, Mum's face changes again. She looks younger, forthright, about to deliver an important utterance. Her lips are pursed, her eyes determined.

'I'm sorry too,' says Mum. Then, as temperamental as an April day in England, her face dissolves into helplessness again and her eyes tip over with tears and she sniffles. The phone is wrenched away and then it's Shirl's face again and she's not happy.

'It really isn't on, waltzing back into our lives again as if no time has passed.'

The usual rant from bitter Shirl. Then I hear Mum's voice again.

She says, 'But, Shirley, isn't that exactly what you can do with family?'

Shirl looks annoyed then barks down the phone, 'We're busy making lunch. Try another time. Bye.'

And they're gone.

How was your call? WhatsApp asks me.

I say aloud, 'Not good.' Then I add, 'But it wasn't that bad either.'

I know it's been my fault for drawing away from them since they went so far away after Dad's death. I tell myself I'm going to start messaging Shirley every week from now on. And I'm going to ask to speak to Mum more often too. Whatever bullshit, silliness and outright lies I've found in this wellness kick, there's one very important thing it's done for me: it's made me take tentative steps back towards my family, who I've felt alienated from for so long. It's hard to do . . . but it feels good. It feels worth it. As Clio said, change is painful.

Chapter 16

It's Thursday evening, the night before the wellness weekend retreat begins and I'm ridiculously excited. I've already packed my bags which are ready and waiting at the end of my bed. I'll be driving there tomorrow straight from work as I'm such an eager beaver to get there. Yes, I am going on the retreat, despite the fact that the cost is . . . eye-watering. It's £1600 for two nights. Jeeeeezus. I could go on a fabulous fortnight somewhere glamorous and hot for that. It's crazy money, I know it is. But . . . I couldn't resist. When do I ever treat myself? Hardly ever, that's what. And those savings of mine sitting there waiting for a rainy day . . . ?

Before that though I'm on my way to meet Jacqui for a drink at her local pub. We're going to talk about how her wellness articles are going and I'll be giving her more material for it after the retreat. It's all coming together nicely. I haven't seen Jacqui for a bit as we've both been so busy, so I'm looking forward to seeing my bestie. I park up and sprint through the car park to avoid the pelting rain and arrive in the bar out of breath and damp. I find Jacqui sitting in a little booth in the next room. It's one of those old pubs that has two rooms at either end of the bar, perhaps one for the men and one for the women. I actually wouldn't mind that being reinstituted, to be honest. I'm not much to look at but Jacqui is and when we're in pubs it's tedious how regularly some bloke or two will come over and try to talk to us while we're clearly busy and not interested. The arrogant confidence of some men never ceases to amaze me, that they're so utterly convinced of their attractiveness that they can't comprehend that you don't want to talk to them and just want them to leave you the fuck alone. Dad used to call these types of men the 'cocksures'. *Tell those cocksures to bugger off*, he'd say to me and Jacqui when he'd drop us off at a pub in our late teens. I hope there are no cocksures tonight, as I'm buzzing with excitement and I really don't need some idiot man killing my vibe.

I arrive at Jacqui's booth and cry, 'Jac!' in our customary way. But no shouting of 'Lu!' is forthcoming. Jacqui glances up and gives me a weak smile. I lean over to give her a hug. Despite looking fabulous as ever, with a suede jacket that looks like she stole it from a rodeo, plus her hair plaited round her head like a Swiss milkmaid, she looks truly fed up.

'What's up?' I say, taking a quick sip of the gin and tonic she's already bought for me, my favourite pub tipple. Just one tonight, I tell myself, as I'm driving plus I want to be fresh for tomorrow. 'Thanks for this.'

'My fucking boss shelved my wellness articles idea.'

'Oh no!' I cry. 'Why would he do that?'

'He said wellness used to be a big thing but it's not very zeitgeisty right now. It's absolute bollocks! There are two TV

177

dramas on streaming right now about wellness plus loads of podcasts about it. He's talking crap.'

She looks so downhearted. I'm mad on her behalf.

'Can't you tell this idiot all that?'

'I did! But he wasn't interested. He said local people don't care what's streaming on TV or on podcasts. They want to know what's happening with parking permits and whether the swimming pool is going to be refurbished. They don't want to think about national trends or serious stuff. They read our paper for an escape from all that.'

'That sounds like bollocks to me,' I say. 'Just because it's a local paper, doesn't mean it's got to dumb down.'

'Well, he disagrees. He keeps reminding me that the average reading ability of a local paper reader is much lower than you'd think and we have to keep it simple. I keep telling him that I can still write an interesting article on an interesting topic yet keep the prose relatively simple. But he doesn't listen to me. He's such a patronising arsehole, to me and our readers. He told me last week that the best thing about my work is that I have a "nice turn of phrase". Nice . . . isn't *nice* just the fucking pits? I don't want to be "nice". I want to be groundbreaking! I want to be Gloria Steinem! Nellie Bly or Marie Colvin! Bernstein and Woodward! God, Lu, I'm just dying at this job. It's killing me as a writer.'

I reach out and squeeze her hand. 'Oh honey, you are such a brilliant writer. You always were. Back at school you got the literature prize three years running! I've always loved your work. Maybe it's time to move on from the local newspaper business?'

Jacqui shakes her head vigorously. 'Impossible. Barna's cleaning business has lost a couple of big clients recently and so we're not doing too great financially. I can't go freelance. We can't afford it. Plus kids are so fucking expensive. Holly needs new ice skates as her feet seem to be growing like a time-lapse film of a runner bean seedling. Freya is going on a skiing holiday with school that costs an arm and a leg. And Harvey . . . well, Harvey is still ill and not getting any better. All these different aches and pains with his limbs and bruising on his skin and headaches and teeth problems. GP thinks he might have something called EDS. I've been googling it. It's not pretty. Hypermobility. Can cause all sorts of problems all over the body, not just the joints. Waiting lists for consultant rheumatologists are over a year on the NHS. We're looking into taking him private. We don't have any insurance. We'll have to pay for everything. I've no idea if we can afford it or not. It's a bit of a nightmare.'

Oh God, poor darling Jac. The weight of the world is on her shoulders. I think of the ridiculous amount of money I've just spent on this retreat.

'Let me give you the money, darling.'

'Oh, God no! I mean, thanks, but no thanks. Friendship and money don't mix well at all. Not at all. Don't worry, we'll work something out. Barna's mum has a bit put away. She might send us some.'

I take her hand again and squeeze it. 'But I can give it to you right now. For heaven's sake, I've just spent silly money on this wellness retreat bollocks, so the least I can do is pay for my friend's gorgeous son's treatment. How much do you need?'

But Jac shakes her head again. 'Absolutely not. I have my pride left, if nothing else. But thank you. Look, I'm sick of the sound of my own voice talking about my miserable woes. Tell me about this weekend. Tell me everything. I just want to listen to you bang on about its nonsense. It'll cheer me up.'

'I'd rather talk about how we can start sorting some of your problems,' I tell her. 'Tell me more about this EDS condition that Harvey might have.'

'Honestly, I can't bear to, if that's okay. I just want to escape it all for one night. Tell me about this Clarity with Clio retreat thing.'

Jacqui is determined, I can see that. I want to help her so badly. I wish I had a magic wand.

'Well, okay. If that's what you really want. It starts tomorrow night. The first night is a kind of marketplace event where there are loads of stalls and you can peruse and buy stuff if you want. The Saturday involves one two-hour group session with Clio in the morning, then another in the afternoon. The rest of the day you can wander the grounds or go to other treatments and classes, like yoga and massage and stuff with other practitioners. Then on Sunday there are one-to-one sessions with Clio in the morning, then lunch, then that's it.'

'Sounds quite full-on,' says Jacqui. 'What are the classes about?'

'I can't remember all the descriptions. Here, have a look at the website.'

I get it up on my phone and show her Clio's dedicated webpage for the retreat, which she runs every year.

'My God, it's at Roseland Hall. Remember that snobby cow from school – urgh, what was her name? The one who said her fiancé gave her an engagement ring that was just "chippings"?'

'Bitsy Sheridan?'

'Yes! Bitsy! Short for Elizabeth. And all her friends and family called her Bitsy for some godforsaken reason and we secretly called her Bitchy.'

'Ha ha! Yes! What about her?'

'Her parents bloody own Roseland Hall. They bought it off some bankrupted gentry a few years back. They live in an annex and rent the rest out for conferences and this wellness kind of thing. They must be minting it. I mean, how much was it for the weekend?'

I feel embarrassed all of a sudden, though I never usually am with Jacqui.

'Too much money to reveal. I can't even believe I paid it.'

'What? Tell me! It's not like you to be coy.'

'More than £1500,' I say and grimace. Now I feel really dumb to have paid that money, especially when Jacqui is struggling so much.

Her face says it all. Blank surprise.

'Wow . . . ' is all she says. I feel really uncomfortable now.

'Yeah . . . ' is all I can think of to say.

'But . . . Lu, that's a hell of a price tag just to impress your bosses.'

'Oh, I'm not going on the retreat to impress them, not really.'

Jacqui looks nonplussed and I'm starting to feel a bit defensive.

'Well . . . why are you going then? I thought you hated all this wellness bullshit.'

'I do, I mean, all the other wellness bullshit. But Clio isn't like that.'

Jacqui looks curiously at me. 'We talked about your first

181

session with her. That sounded like it went well. But you haven't told me any more about further sessions with her. What were they like?'

I'm excited to explain it to Jacqui because I haven't really said much to her about it, as she's been so busy. And strangely, I've kind of wanted to keep it to myself. I know that something miraculous has been happening with Clio. But it's really hard to explain it to someone else, even my best friend.

'She's . . . I don't know how to explain it really. She's changed my life. After that first session, I went back to my childhood with my dad. Fuck, it was so moving, you know? Seeing him again so young. It was . . . incredible. And then last time, I went into my own mother's head, when we were little. It made me see everything from her point of view, how hard it was being a mother. I rang New Zealand after and spoke to my mum on video call. Just felt totally different about her this time. Honestly, I do think my sessions with Clio are changing my life. *She's* changing my life. And she's had cancer. And went into remission using nutrition when she decided to give up the chemo. And I've got my boss to agree to having her as the keynote speaker at the staff conference. Clio is amazing, honestly!'

Whenever I'd usually explain something great that's happening in my life to Jacqui, she'd be right on board and celebrating my wins with me. Maybe it's because she's preoccupied with her own troubles, or maybe . . . I don't know. But her face just looks concerned, not pleased. And she's not saying anything.

'What?' I ask, still all lit up from talking about Clio. But Jacqui's face is throwing a shadow on everything.

'Have you drunk the Kool-Aid or what?'

There's that cynical face of Jacqui's I usually love, when we rip the shit out of some pretentious nonsense. But she doesn't understand.

'No, no. It's not like that. Clio isn't like that. You'd understand if you met her. She's the genuine article. She's helped me come up with all these incredible insights into my relationships. I couldn't have done that without her. It's like she can read my mind!'

Jacqui leans back in her chair and finishes off her customary negroni.

'Do you want another drink? My round,' I say, polishing off my G&T. I'll get a simple slimline tonic next, I think.

'No, I don't,' says Jacqui, shockingly turning down a drink, which she never does. 'I want to talk to you about this Clio bullshit.'

Now I'm annoyed.

'Hey, it's not bullshit. Honestly, Jac, you just have to be there to understand it.'

Jacqui laughs scoffingly. 'No, I don't. I've heard this nonsense before. She cured her own cancer? That doesn't happen, Lu! It never does! Drinking juice cleanses to wash out cancerous toxins and all that shite? This is dangerous stuff! And all this mind-reading she seems to be doing on you? Don't forget you filled out a highly extensive questionnaire about your life before you started. That's how these grifters work. They harvest information from you, work out your weaknesses and exploit them. And now you've not only given her nearly two grand of your own money, you've let her inveigle her way into your work life too. You're so smart, Lu! I can't believe you can't see it!'

The whole time Jacqui is talking, I can feel my annoyance

rising, turning into indignation and now I'm really pissed off with her.

'It's not like that!' I cry. 'I am smart, yes. You know that. I wouldn't be taken in by a charlatan. Clio is the real deal. She hasn't asked me for anything. She just offers things and then it's up to me if I want to take part in it. And it was me who asked her to be the keynote speaker, not the other way round. Look, why don't you let me book a session with her for you? I bet she could help you with your issues right now, help you see things more clearly.'

Jacqui is shaking her head at me now. 'God, no. I'd rather lick a nettle than let that woman loose in my mind. Listen, darling, you know I love you. I always want the best for you. But this kind of therapy, it can be so dangerous, with someone unhinged like this . . . '

'She's not unhinged!' I cry.

'Bloody hell, you're so defensive of her,' says Jacqui, shocked. 'This is a really bad sign, chick. She's got you exactly where she wants you. Spending money like water, listening to every damn word, letting her in to every aspect of your life. It's really bloody worrying, Lu. Can't you see it? Can't you be objective about it, for one moment? You sound like a giddy schoolgirl, for fuck's sake. This really isn't like you.'

Now I'm enraged. 'Well, maybe I've changed,' I spit out at Jacqui. 'And . . . and actually . . . there's no maybe about it. I *have* changed. I *am* changing. And maybe you don't like that. Maybe you just want me to stay the same as I always was. Poor, lonely Lucy, always there for you because I have no life. Maybe it wouldn't suit you if I actually found myself and changed my life. Maybe I won't be there at your beck and call anymore and you don't like that.'

Jesus Christ, I've never spoken to Jacqui like that before. I have no idea where that came from. But she was attacking something that means a lot to me. Someone who means a lot to me. I can't have that, oldest friend or no. I'm breathless from my tirade and wipe my eyes and take a deep breath to recover. Then I look up at Jacqui's face.

'Fuck you, Lu.'

She shoves the table to the side, throws her handbag over her shoulder and leaves.

Chapter 17

Change is painful. That's what Clio said. That's what I keep telling myself as I look at my phone to see that Jacqui hasn't answered any of my messages from last night or today. I've apologised. I've tried to explain. But no reply. I hate this. Jacqui and I never fall out. But . . . change is painful. And maybe Jac needs to change too, to see me differently. Hopefully, that's all it'll take, for her to accept the change in me and embrace me as I am. I've texted enough. I won't text again, until she replies. Which will be soon. I'm sure it will. Jacqui won't stay mad at me for long. She never has.

I rush through my Friday and leave bang on home time, driving over to Roseland Hall, in the heart of the High Weald countryside, the evening fast falling into darkness. I turn off the winding B road to the long driveway of the hall. I can see the hall through the trees, like a wellness version of Manderley. My stomach starts churning. I'm nervous. I don't know why I'm nervous, not really. I can do small talk when I need to. I didn't know how to dress for this retreat though.

I ordered some yoga pants and other activewear from M&S a few days back and ended up returning most of it, because honestly I felt I looked a twat in all of them. I'm just not an activewear type of person. I felt like a fraud. So I've brought a few pairs of leggings and some baggy T-shirts for the sessions. That will do, surely. Clio's usual class doesn't require any kind of special clothing but the website says something about gentle floor exercises so I'm coming prepared. Plus I bring a ton of other stuff for the socialising bits. Today I'm wearing some comfy jeans and a stripy top and jacket. I'm trying to go for smart casual. I realise I'm nervous because this isn't work and it isn't socialising – it's somewhere in between and I'm not comfortable there. Anyway, hey-ho, here we go. I've pulled up in the extensive car park. My Ford Focus looks entirely out of place amidst the Audis and BMWs and Range Rovers and even a couple of Aston Martins. I am not rich enough to mix with these people. I start to regret spending that £1600 on this. But then, I wouldn't be part of Clio's special weekend and I really wanted that. I really want to see what else she has to offer. She's helped me so much already, not only to reconnect with my family but to reconnect with myself too. It's all worth it.

I bring my suitcase in bumpily as it trips over the pebbled driveway up to the front door of the hall. A woman in perfect make-up, razor-sharp bobbed hair and pencil skirt, holding a clipboard, smiles broadly as I drag my case up the steps. I know I've packed far too much stuff for two nights. But I had no idea what to bring or what not to bring, so I brought my entire wardrobe instead. The woman watches me struggle and keeps grinning. Finally, I get my case up onto the top step.

'Well done!' she says, hinting I suppose that my suitcase is ridiculously large for two nights. Don't fucking baggage-shame me, woman! That's what I want to cry. But I don't, of course. 'Good evening and welcome to Clarity with Clio weekend wellness retreat!' she says. Wow, she's got so much make-up on, she looks like Aunt Sally.

'Hi,' I say, puffed.

'Can I please take your surname?'

'Cooper.'

She riffles through the pages attached to the clipboard for what seems like an age. She's frowning and then riffles through the entire lot again. I start to doubt that I've even booked a place or paid all that money. But it's definitely disappeared from my account, leaving a huge hole. So my name must be on there somewhere. This always seems to happen to me. My name never seems to be on the right lists. I can never arrive at any event with confidence. Imposter syndrome. After an age, the woman says, 'Ms Lucy Cooper?'

Urgh, at last.

'Yes!'

'Marvellous. Please go through these double doors and to reception on the right where you can check in. The wellness mart has already begun in the main hall, so do make your way down there when you've settled in.'

'It's already begun?' I say, anxiously.

'Ah, please don't worry. The mart is an event running throughout the weekend, where stallholders are awaiting your interest. There is no formal time to attend, as you can visit at any time. Please, do settle yourself in your room first and come down when you are ready. There is a buffet provided from 6pm in the same hall which will be replenished until

9pm, so you are welcome to come down at any time to eat and browse. Enjoy your Clarity with Clio weekend!'

That's my cue to bugger off, as more people are coming up the steps behind me. I turn to see three women about my age all giggling together and talking about cocktails. Doesn't sound very wellness-y to me (although I could murder a cocktail about now). I go through the doors into the stone-tiled floor of Roseland Hall's foyer. Huge flower arrangements on pillars on either side, a cupola through which you can see the night sky speckled with stars above and on my right, the reception desk with another clone of clipboard woman. She even has the same ironed hair.

The gaggle of women are coming up behind me, as I go through check-in and finally I get to escape to my room. It's on the ground floor along a long dim corridor with a door at the end decorated with stained glass. It's all terribly nice here. Despite the cost and my nerves, I'm glad I've come. It's an experience and different from my usual weekends. I tell myself I'm going to dump my stuff in my room but not hide there. I'm going to get down to the 'wellness mart' thing and get some food, because I'm starving.

The room is also terribly nice. Clean, small, perfectly formed. Bath with shower over. I don't have a bath in my house, so I plan on taking advantage of that later with the complimentary bubble bath. Okay, so, here I go, shutting my door and making my way down the long corridor of doom to the weekend of peopley small talk with people . . . urgh. PEOPLE. Even the word breaks me out in hives. But I can do this. I must do this. Because I've spent too much money to hide away in my bathroom. You might be thinking, how is this woman so nervous about small talk with strangers when her literal job is organising people? Well, you see, at work I have a mask on. Not literally. But I have a work persona, honed from years of interaction with colleagues in mostly tricky situations. Yet somewhere like this, doing something like this, there is no mask. I'm not my work self. I'm just myself. And the honest truth is I'm not all that comfortable just being myself. Except home alone. Or when I used to be with Dad. Or with Jacqui . . . (I check my phone again. Still no reply from Jac. But I can't think about that right now.)

In the foyer I'm directed to the wellness mart in the main hall by a handy sign on a stand and as I approach, the hubbub of sound increases with every step, as do my nerves. Finally, I'm in the main hall and it's absolutely bloody packed. I pause briefly in the doorway and scan the crowd of people milling around the stalls to see if Clio is there and I can say hello to her. I think I'll feel better if I know at least one person here, but I can't see her anywhere. I can't stand in this doorway forever. Okay, here we go. I'm going to stroll in a leisurely manner around the stalls and look like I have purpose. I know you want to know about all the stalls in this temple to wellness. And let me tell you, if you're looking for the height of wellness bullshit, you will not be disappointed. I know that Clio is totally legit. But I'm surprised to find that the businesses she has chosen to come and tout their wares here this weekend sound like a list of cautionary tales against wellness scams.

Ready? These are the things you can buy, if you so wish to waste your hard-earned cash:

Earthing shoes – I asked the lady and she said they have metals in the soles which allow you to connect with healing electrical energy from the ground and this will cure your sleeplessness, reduce pain and help any wounds to heal more quickly. Okayyyyy . . . I want the science on this, I tell her. She says this is beyond science. But has been proven by 'anecdotal evidence'. There's that phrase again . . . I mean, I like the idea, of earthing, of being in connection with the ground. But . . . electrical charges healing my wounds? Her cheapest pair costs £170. I could stick my toes in a plug socket for free.

Moonjuice – typical grifty drinks, potions and lotions at exorbitant prices. I'm sure they do help (the owner of the company make millions off your gullibility).

Glitter smoothies – don't even start.

Crystal-infused water bottle – shut up.

Charcoal lattes – the guy at the stall tells me they are also called goth lattes due to their stunning appearance. He tells me that the drink will 'remove toxins from your body and eliminate disease'. Which disease? I ask him. A wide range, he replies. He wants to give me a sample. 'Charcoal lattes can affect the absorption of birth control pills. Are you on birth control?' he asks. I reply, deadpan, 'Do I *look* like I'm on birth control?' That was the end of our conversation.

Sleep tents – I mean, isn't that the point of tents? This one is something to do with sensory blackout. Okay, that actually sounds appealing. I can't afford the £457 price tag though, not after splurging on this whole weekend.

Goop jade yoni eggs – all you need to know is that you shove it up your hoo-ha. I hope these ones aren't second-hand. I saw a second-hand dildo for sale on Facebook Marketplace once.

Raw milk – urgh.

Bovine colostrum supplements – double urgh.

Personalised vitamins – I could get a Sharpie and write my

name on a multivitamin and it'd have more of a personalised effect, I bet.

Aura photography – no.

Bee sting therapy – also no.

Oxygen bars – you stick something over your face and get a purer oxygen dose for £75 a hit. I can get my oxygen for free actually. It's called breathing.

Dumb phones – digital detox. No Smartphone capabilities. Just tapping the same damn button four times to get the letter you want, like back in the nineties. Oh and some retro games. All a very good idea, I'm sure. But I know I'm addicted to my phone and honestly, life is hard and it gives me joy to scroll through idiotic shit on Facebook so, no thanks.

Adaptogenic drinks – the couple selling these tell me they can reduce anxiety. Any side effects? I ask. Can cause diarrhoea. So, I would swap feeling worried for the raging shits. Great.

Lion's Mane coffee – mushroom coffee. Two words that should never go together in a sentence.

Ear seeds – just fuck off.

Do any of them have positive effects? Mayyybe. Who knows? Placebo effect? Or real effect? Nobody knows. But the crazy price tag of every single one of these is a red flag. I'm really surprised that Clio has let these charlatans into her weekend retreat. I mean, isn't she against all this nonsense? I suppose she has to make a living though and I bet these folk pay a good rate for their pitches. There are plenty more stalls than my selection here and I've done all of them now and I'm feeling nervous again. Then I see the buffet over by the far wall behind the stalls and I realise how hungry I still am.

I make my way over there and see a veritable sea of bowls

of healthy-looking stuff I really don't want to eat. Oh shit, it's a wellness retreat isn't it . . . that means no real food. Apparently, according to a large cardboard sign, it's all 'vegan, organic, minimal processing, free from artificial flavourings and colours, sweetener-free, no trans fat, no added salt, no corn syrup and sugar-free.' Free from all the fun things. Okay, I'm really hungry so here goes. I spoon a bunch of salads onto my plate and they do look pretty – rainbow foods and all that – but I could murder a bacon sandwich right now. Or a kebab. But I'm trying to be positive about this. After all, it really would be a good idea to reduce my intake of wildly unhealthy foods and maybe change my old ways a bit by trying something new. And trying to be positive. And also I'm trying to decide what gelatinous substance is in this cold stir fry bowl I'm poking at with a spoon – tofu? Jackfruit? – as it looks deeply unappetising.

'It's called seitan,' says a voice behind me and I look round. A woman around the same age as me, with long blonde hair pulled up into a bouncy ponytail on the top of her head, wearing pink and grey activewear from head to toe and looking somewhat condescendingly at me . . . and I know her. I know that face from my past. Who the hell is it? Come on, post-menopausal brain, you slow fucker. 'It's wheat gluten, in case you have issues with soya beans. But if you have issues with gluten, then you should avoid. I helped Clio with the food choices for the weekend. I teach yoga here, so you can sign up for my class if you like.'

Oh. My. God.

It's Bitchy Sheridan. The one whose parents own Roseland Hall. The snobby cow I went to school with. Jacqui will just DIE if I send her a pic of this one.

'Why, it's you!' I cry and throw my arms around Bitchy. I know she hasn't clocked at all who I am. I know I'm unrecognisable from the old days. I had dyed purple hair and a massive fringe to hide my face the last time she saw me. In fact, my fringe was so big, I doubt Bitchy Sheridan has ever actually seen my face at all.

When we come up for air, Bitchy is looking at me like I'm nuts.

'Hey . . . you!' she tries. Her discomfort is delicious. You might think it's bitchy calling her Bitchy. And you'd be right. But she really was a nasty piece of work at school. She called me Doughnut Dinah, after the shop in town (Donut Diner) where she saw me once getting a large bag for my family which she told everyone was just for me. I never lived it down and that name stuck with me for the last four years of secondary school. So yeah, I pretty much hate her.

'How the devil are you, Bitsy?'

'Erm . . . I'm good! I'm so good! I love teaching my yoga classes. They are very spiritual, you know. I incorporate a range of techniques to stretch both body and mind, allowing you to connect with your most feminine essence. They really are the best workout you can ask for, especially at our age as older post-menopausal women kicking the world's ass right now. We are warriors! So, you really should come. You know what though, I'm so busy this weekend, I don't have time to talk right now. Could you give me your business card and I'll get back to you later?'

She's hoping I'll give her something with my name on it. I do have business cards, actually, right here in my inside pocket. I always carry a few around. But there's no way she's getting her hands on one.

'I don't have one, sorry, Bitsy. It's so good to see you! Remember that time we smashed the badminton record together? Happy days!'

Bitchy played badminton but I never played it. I couldn't hit a moving thing to save my life. I'm just winding her up and it's so much fun.

'Oh . . . yeah! That was so . . . fab! You were a . . . veritable wizard with a shuttlecock!'

'Thanks, Bitsy!' I cry and grin fiendishly at her as she wilts visibly. 'Oh Bitsy. Could we do a quick selfie I can send to our old pals Miranda and Camilla and Bunty and Cunty?'

I hold my phone up while she's still reeling at Cunty. And take a snap. Jacqui will fucking love this!

Bitchy extricates herself. 'Must be off! Things to . . . do and such!'

And off she goes, confused and flustered. Ha ha haaaaaaaa! That's made my day.

I go on Messenger and look at all the unanswered messages to Jac. Well, she can't ignore this one. I press send on the selfie we just took.

'Hello there, Lucy,' says a voice beside me. Has Bitchy remembered me by some vague chance?

I look up and who should I see standing there but our very favourite frenemy, Tara Harryman. She's here too? Clio invited *her* to be in her special, exclusive group?

Chapter 18

My nemesis, Tara. She's wearing relatively normal clothes compared to most of the activewear-obsessed women delegates here (and yes, they are all women, not a single man). Tara has a relaxed grey T-shirt tucked into dark grey cords with sparkly high-top trainers on. She looks really cool. Wish I could be effortlessly cool. Unfortunately, my whole life I've been uncool despite lashings of effort.

And she wastes no time in going straight in for the attack.

'Taking this wellness lie a little too far, aren't you, Lucy?'

'It's not a lie,' I reply indignantly. 'I happen to think Clio is marvellous, which is why she's going to be keynote speaker for us.'

'Yes, I know she agreed. I had a word with her about it too.'

If I were a cartoon character, there would be steam coming out of my ears.

'Well, you didn't need to, Tara. She said yes straight away to me.'

Tara smiles her little smug smile at me, as if to say she

knows she can get to me so easily and I always bite. I need to be more cool, calm and collected with her, like she is.

'So, Tara,' I say, changing my tone to feign interest. 'Tell me what you're looking forward to this weekend.'

'Only Clio's sessions, to be honest,' says Tara, glancing around the hall. 'Most of the rest of this wellness stuff they've got here is pretentious bollocks. Expensive pretentious bollocks.'

'You're not wrong,' I say, loath to agree with her.

'I mean, I'm a bit surprised there's so much woo-woo stuff here, as Clio has always said to me how much she's against the worst kind of wellness rubbish. But I had a chat with one of the stallholders and she said Clio gets a commission on their fee. So I suppose a gal has to make a living.'

'Well, yes. I'm guessing it's expensive to hire out Roseland Hall and she has to get her money back in a range of ways, I suppose.'

Tara hunches her shoulders and her eyes flit around the room.

'It's just awful stuff here though, isn't it? Which is your best worst product you've seen here tonight? Mine was ear seeds. How on earth can a "twenty-four-carat plated ion seed" – whatever the hell an "ion seed" is anyway – that you glue on your ear to detox and nourish yourself or whatever – how can that have any damn effect on your body or mind? Absolute rubbish.'

'Well, yes!' I can't disagree with her. As she talks to me, she's eyeing the crowd in that way people do when they're looking for someone more interesting to talk to. 'If you'd rather talk to literally anyone else than me, Tara, then please go ahead. I have a plate of rabbit food to devour.'

'I don't know a soul here,' she replies and sighs. 'Only you. And Clio. Some yoga woman accosted me and tried to persuade me to come to her sessions. Her ponytail bobbed backwards and forwards as she harangued me about accessing my most feminine self. My God, the woman would not take no for an answer. I mean, I like yoga. It's great for your body. But the teacher has to have the right vibe. This woman would drive me nuts. I didn't think yoga bullies existed but there you go. I saw you throw your arms around her. Old friend? Family?'

I could see she wanted to get one over on me that way, so I feel like stringing her along, but honestly, I'm so tired and hungry that I can't actually be bothered.

'I knew her at school and couldn't stand her. She didn't recognise me so I made out we were best friends and badminton champions together, just to watch her squirm.'

I shrug and go back to filling my plate.

Tara laughs and says, 'Lucy, I didn't realise you were so devious! Christ, I knew girls at school like her too. They were always called Allegra or Minty or something.'

'She's called Bitsy.'

Tara looks at me and we both burst out laughing.

'I know!' I say, still laughing.

'Well, look. I don't know anyone here and there's no sign of Clio. It's like milling around at a wedding when the only person you know is the bride. Absolutely deadly. I'm going to hide in my room.'

'Okay,' I say, a bit speechless as I never expected to have a conversation like this with my frenemy.

Tara hesitates before leaving. 'Listen,' she says. 'Obviously we're work rivals and all that. And there's a lot on the line.

But how about . . . how about we call a truce for the weekend, just to make everything a bit easier here? What do you say?'

I'm surprised but also relieved. I don't want the whole weekend ruined by animosity bubbling away and threatening to boil over. That is not the vibe I expected or wanted from this retreat.

'I say aye. Here's to a temporary armistice.'

'Excellent. See you tomorrow at Clio's thing.'

And off she goes to avoid people. Just like I tend to do. Maybe we have more in common than I thought.

It's actually a shame that we hate each other so much as it turns out she's quite easy to talk to. When I get my promotion and we're not in direct competition anymore, maybe I'll chat with her again and we'll get on okay, who knows? For now, I'll just need to avoid her as much as possible. The more she knows about me, the more she can exploit. Knowledge is power, after all.

I go and sit on one of the chairs lining the hall to eat my rabbit food. It tastes okay, not too bad. A bit of spice and different textures. I scroll on my phone to ward off sad loser vibes, while everyone else in this room talks to each other like they've shared organs for transplants. It occurs to me that I'm always the one in a group that seems to know nobody, while other people all seem to have had an alert to meet up and get friendly, while I never had that memo. I eat as quickly as I can then head off to my room, like sensible Tara did. Wish I'd stayed up there all evening, to be honest. I get into the bath and wonder why the hell I'm here. But it's okay. It'll all be worth it once I'm in Clio's sessions.

I look at my phone. No reply from Jacqui to my pic of me and Bitsy, though I can see that she's seen it. I sigh. I miss my friend.

After an early night and an early rise in the morning, I'm fresh and ready for breakfast. I don't see Tara at breakfast nor Clio. I haven't seen Clio yet at all. Maybe she stays in her room and orders room service, like a celebrity, to avoid the crush. And I bet there would be a crush with all these women fan-girling over Clio. It makes me feel a bit weird, actually, that I have so much regard for someone and everyone else here does too, but I push the thought to the back of my mind. I've not been in that situation before, but this is different, I tell myself. I'm usually rooting for the underdog and hate the popular types. Breakfast is actually nice, despite no fry up or pastries. There's lots of fresh fruit and nuts and seeds and yoghurt, so I make up a bowl like I have done at home and it tastes good. The rooibos tea – which seemed the least weird of all the teas on offer – tastes good too. This healthy eating thing can be okay, sometimes. Though a fried egg sandwich about now wouldn't go amiss. I look down at my baggy T-shirt and leggings again and feel uncool and unlike every other cool person in this place. Oh well, nothing I can do. Maybe I should've bought some earthing shoes. Actually, maybe fucking not.

Today – Saturday – involves one two-hour group session with Clio in the morning, then another in the afternoon. Between classes, you can do what you like; there are other classes to sign up for in between and all evening (including Bitsy's yoga – no thanks) plus you can go for a walk outside, if the rain ever stops, that is. It's pissing it down out there.

Finally, after another little sojourn in my room after breakfast awaiting the right time, 9am comes and I make my way to the other side of reception for the first of Clio's sessions. As I approach the room, I can hear the hubbub from within which makes me nervous again. In you go, Lucy Cooper. You have every right to be here, my internal monologue tells me. My internal monologue is usually a right bitch. My God, the things she says to me, I wouldn't say to my worst enemy. But today, she's feeling positive, heavily influenced by the excitement of seeing Clio again. Come on, then. Let's do this.

Inside is a studio with mirrors along one wall and about twenty or so women arranged in haphazard lines chatting away to each other, sitting on yoga mats. Oh shit, I didn't bring a yoga mat. Did it say to bring one? I feel such an idiot. Then I see there are a bunch of them hanging up at the back, the same colours as the ones the women are using. Why do I always assume I'm the idiot? I really do need to give myself a break. As I walk over to collect one, I see Tara over the other side of the room with no gaps near her. I mean, I wasn't going to sit near her, obviously, as she's my enemy. But I have to admit it would be nice to talk to someone I know, even her. I find a spot, but it's not quite big enough so I have to ask two women to shove their yoga mats up slightly, to which request I'm given looks that suggest I just asked to piss on their fish and chips. At last, I can sit down on my mat. I don't have my phone so I can't disappear into that. I have to sit there and watch all these women talking to each other and laughing and bonding and I can't think of a damn thing to say to anyone. Sometimes the loneliest place to be is surrounded by other people. I'm gazing around the room wondering how all these people do it, so effortlessly. Then, Tara catches my eye and rolls her eyes so far back, she could give herself a brain haemorrhage. I laugh and the two women beside me look at me with alarm. They must think there's a madwoman in their midst, sitting alone, laughing at nothing and not even wearing proper yoga pants or a skin-tight bra top. And at that moment, when I feel suitably chastised by the cool women around me marking me out as the uncool loser, Clio walks into the room.

Everyone lets out a collective gasp when she comes in and then an instant hush. She's wearing pretty casual stuff, navy blue leggings and a sleeveless top, her grey bob perfectly bobbing as she walks. But it's not about what she looks like, it's just her . . . Clio. She has that aura about her. Christ, I can't believe I used the word aura. I mean, I don't believe in visible ones, that you can photograph or draw with crayons. But some people definitely have an invisible aura about them that everyone can sense. It's a kind of . . . luminosity, if you know what I mean. Something I know I've definitely never possessed in my life. I'm so aura-less I may as well be transparent. But Clio has it in spades. She kneels down on a yoga mat on a raised platform in front of the mirrors. Everyone is silent.

'Hello campers,' says Clio in a deadpan way through her microphone and everyone laughs. It's like we needed permission to make a sound. There's a kind of reverence in the air and I'm totally up for that too. Everyone in this room thinks she's the bee's knees. Before she walked in, I felt utterly lost in this sea of well-dressed women but now Clio is here I feel utterly connected to them all. Clio brings us all together somehow. It's a wonderful feeling and something I don't think I've felt for a long time, if ever.

'Thank you all for coming today and for the whole weekend. It's such a great feeling to see you all here together. My practice being one-to-one means that I've got to know all of you as individuals, so an opportunity like this is just marvellous to me, to see all of these wonderful women together in the same room. I hope you've been getting to know each other as I just know you will all find allies and comrades and sisters in this room, if you try. The power in this room right now is . . . well, it's given me quite the shiver. It's an awesome power from each and every one of you, truly. I can feel it coming off you in waves. I love that.'

Clio looks down to her feet and smiles, then rearranges herself into a crossed-legged position. Everyone else does this too, as if from a silent signal. She's right. There is a power in this room. It's the weirdest thing. It's as if she's aimed it all at us and we're reflecting it right back. I've never felt anything quite like it. It is vibrant.

'So, you're all familiar with my past-life regression therapy. We're going to do something a bit different today to open your minds, also using our physical selves to open ourselves up to everything we need from the world. You know me by now. You know I don't believe in much of the wellness brouhaha we're bombarded with on Instagram and Facebook. There's far too much mendacity in the world. What I want our space here to be is one free from nonsense, from bullshit, from the endless chatter of social media but also from our own minds. It's not about emptying your minds though. I believe our minds can be our friends, if we stop treating them like our enemies. Today I want you to reach out and embrace that inner voice, as if it were your own self as a child. And that's where we're going to start today. Please close your eyes and get as comfortable as you can in your cross-legged position. If your knees are bothering you or the hard floor under your bum doesn't feel great, then feel free to sit another way. What we want to avoid is lying down, as we want to be in a calm, relaxed posture but wide awake. For we have work to do.'

A handful of women shift positions but I feel okay with crossed legs for the moment, so I stay where I am. Thankfully, Clio has not put on any yoga-y type music that's supposed to relax you but I always find myself analysing it to work out why it's so shit. I hate that type of music that's supposed to be like white noise or whatever because it never is. It's always big spaced-out synth chords with plinkety-plonk piano chords and it's fucking annoying. So I'm very glad Clio has decided on silence. I'm fine with silence, me. It's comforting.

'You're in a peaceful place and you are alone there. It's a beautiful place. Where is it . . . exactly? Allow your mind to form that beautiful place. A safe place where you feel purely content. I'll wait a moment until you are fully in this place that is real and whole in every particular.'

I'm already in mine. It's near the bridge where I went as a child but it's downriver from there. Somewhere Dad took us – me and Shirl – where we went on a long riverside walk to give Mum some peace and quiet. It was a bend in the river, where a weeping willow tree hung over its bank on the other side, trailing its leaves in the water. Gosh, it was the most beautiful place I've ever been. It's in my mind again. I can almost hear the babbling brook. I can see swallows dipping and rising in the blue sky above, the long branches of the willow gently swaying in a slight breeze. It felt like heaven that time we saw it. It feels like heaven now.

Clio continues, 'In that place, in the distance you'll see a small figure. They are standing alone, waiting. Find them in that place and focus on that small figure. You realise as you watch this figure that it is a child. Look at the child now.'

The child in my mind is standing under a tree in a field on

the opposite side of the river. It's a girl in an A-line skirt with a T-shirt and dark hair. She's watching me, I can tell.

'The child is all alone,' says Clio. 'Cross whatever space lies between you, but walk slowly and gently, as there is no urgency, no drama. The child is waiting for you patiently.'

I look down at the river. Its depths are murky and the water runs quickly so I'm too afraid to step into it. But I must reach the child under the tree. I have to. I look down and see I'm barefoot. I sit on the river bank and slide my feet into the water and it's not long before they find the riverbed. The water is cool and the bed feels solid. No squelchy mud here. It's more like sand but firm. This gives me courage and I cross the stream easily, finding steps in the grass that lead up the other bank. When I reach the top, the little girl under the tree smiles shyly. Oh God, I can see her face now. And I know the exact photo that child is from. It's when I was five, standing on a beach in Torquay holding on to my mum's skirt. I'm wearing a T-shirt with a leaping dolphin on it and a blue chequered gingham skirt. The child is me. I walk across the grassy field until I reach the little girl. She seems happy to see me.

'Look carefully at this child. For however this child appears to you, in whatever form or face it has, you know that the child is you. Let that knowledge rest for a moment. The child is you, your inner child, the child that still lives in all of us. Look at this precious child and remember how we all were back then: full of wonder, curiosity, trust, faith and joy. Reach out to this child now and give that child some comfort, whatever comfort means to you. For the child was all alone. But now there are both of you. And you are together and no longer alone.'

I touch the little girl's hair, a messy bundle of sea-wet hair that's dried in the sun. Mum always cursed my hair when she brushed it as it never lay flat. But I banish that fleeting thought from my head because I only want positive thoughts here. I touch the little girl's face and she beams at me. And then she throws her arms around me and I kneel down to give her the tightest most loving hug I can imagine. We hold on to each other and I can breathe in her hair and sense sea-salt and the tang of seaweed. I loved the beach so much as a child. I loved the sea, the freedom of it, its magnificence. I haven't been to a beach for years. I must go again. God, it feels so good to hold on to her and feel how tightly she loves me and needs me. Oh shit, I'm going to cry.

I don't want to cry in front of these people. I open my eyes to force myself back to reality and realise that quite a few women are crying. There are little sobs here and there and some have tears rolling down their cheeks. It's incredibly moving to see these women give themselves up to the moment and let their emotions leak out of them. I glance over at Tara and her head is nodded down, fallen far forward so it nearly touches her lap. She's lost in the moment. I close my eyes again and the child pulls away and grins at me. Her teeth are gappy and imperfect, her tummy sticking out making her skirt bulge, long dark hairs on her forearms. I see all her imperfections and I love her all the more for them. Maybe this is what it feels like to be a mother: seeing your child's flaws and loving them harder because of them, loving them for their vulnerabilities, not their strengths. I think I would've made a pretty good mother, because I'm a damn cool aunt, I know that. I touch the girl's face and she laughs and skips away, running across the field in pure joy. I let her go. She's happy now.

'You can let your child go on alone now. This child will never be lonely again because now they have you. Inside them, beside them, inside you. You are one. Let them go off into the world and just be themselves. Feel their happiness. Feel their freedom. For it is yours too.'

Chapter 19

Our group session carries on after the inner child bit with some stretching and yoga moves. I've never done much yoga myself. Lots of people talk about it. It's just never appealed to me. But actually, I find I really like the yoga moves we're doing. The moves are strangely energising and relaxing at the same time. We stand up straight, fingers pointing at the ceiling. I can't think of the last time I stretched myself so well. Reminds me of the time I was at a castle dungeon museum somewhere and they showed us a medieval torture rack and I thought to myself that there must've been a few seconds before your limbs dislocated when the rack felt bloody great. We lean down and do this upside-down U shape and lift one leg up and stretch it out. It's warmed me up, I can tell you. Who knew it was such hard work just standing in one spot? It feels really good though. My tired old body feels like it's being used for its real purpose for the first time in years. I mean, I do go for walks. I love walks, especially in ancient places. But work has been so manic the last couple of years that even my walks have gone out of the window. I need to start doing those again. And maybe I'll start doing some yoga too. There's probably stuff on YouTube which would mean I wouldn't have to go to a dreaded class with dreaded people. Anyway, all the yoga stretches go on for a good half-hour or more. I've actually lost track of time, I'm enjoying it so much and the sound of Clio's accompanying voice is so mellow, so smooth, so comforting.

Then, she gets us to all sit cross-legged again on our mats and listen to what's happening now. I feel energised and excited. What else is she going to lead us to? What new wonders next?

'I want to tell you a story, an ancient story.'

Ooh, right up my historical street.

'It's about a ship. A sailing ship that went on a long, long journey far away. It encountered rough seas and storms. Attacks and battles. Sea monsters and encounters with gods and goddesses. Throughout the years of its journey, the ship was damaged here and there. The sailors would use new wood to fix the damage. The ship went through so much on its years' long journey that it needed much new wood to replace the old. So much so, that by the end of its journey, the ship had not one plank of wood remaining from its original form. The ship's very fabric had been completely replaced, by stealth, over time. So, the question is, by the time it came home, was it the same ship?'

I like that. I like that a lot. That's really got me thinking. I mean, it is the same ship, of course it is. The same sailors are on it and it's been through all those adventures. But then again, every single part of it has been replaced. So maybe it isn't the same ship! That's wild.

'I thought you might like that story,' says Clio, smiling at the ripple of interest all around the room. 'And I can see from some of you nodding your heads that you've heard about this ship before. It's the Ship of Theseus, a thought experiment and subject of philosophical debate. Think about it. Is it the same ship? If it isn't, when did it stop being the ship it was? If it is the same ship, what remains of the original ship to make it so? Then think about yourselves. Our bodies regenerate constantly. Cells die, cells are replaced. Our mind receives new material that shapes our thoughts every second of every minute of every hour that we're alive. So, are we the same body that we were? Are we the same mind that we were?'

Wow. That really is mind-blowing. I want to talk about it with someone, hash it out. This is fascinating.

Clio continues, 'I can see that's really got your brains going. Remember we're here this weekend to stretch both your body and your mind. And there's nothing more interesting to the human brain than meeting another human brain. So, I'm going to pair you up with another person in the room. I've decided beforehand which souls in this room will meld well together. I'll read out the names now. Find each other.'

This is a shock. But I'm actually glad to be able to talk to someone. It's been a pretty lonely experience so far, this weekend. And bless Clio, she hasn't left it up to us to make our own pairs. That would be flashbacks to PE lessons as a child and always being the odd one out left to pair up with the teacher, the dreadful embarrassment of that, second only to letting team leaders pick their squad and leaving me till last. Clio has chosen the pairs. I wait with bated breath for my name to be read out.

'Lucy Cooper and Tara Harryman.'

Okay. So, before last night, that would've been my worst nightmare. But the moment Clio says our names, I glance over at Tara and she's grinning at me. She starts to walk over and I'm actually pleased. She is the only one I know here, after all. And I'm finding out she's not such a bitch as I thought too. I'm curious to know her better. Obviously just for competition purposes. I'm not getting soft in my old age. Tara is still the enemy.

But I'm looking forward to discussing this ship idea with her. Whatever one might say about Tara, the truth is she's smart. Really smart. And I admire that.

'Thank God it's you and not some weirdo,' Tara says under her breath and I laugh.

'Yeah and thank God Clio didn't appoint two team leaders to pick and choose in that humiliating ritual from school days.'

'Ha, well, I was the sporty one so I always got to pick.'

'Oh God, you were one of those? Of course you were. Well, I was always the clumsy, chubby one who got left till last.'

Tara says, 'You know what, it was brutal and I bloody hated it when teachers made us do that. I picked the underdogs first, every time.'

'You did not!' I cry. 'I literally don't believe you!'

'Yeah, you're right. I never did. Blame socialisation. I'm a nicer person these days though.'

'Are you though . . . ?' I say and give her a sceptical smile.

'Ha! Probably not. I like you, though, Lucy. You know your shit and you're bloody good at your job. I respect that.'

'I respect that about you too,' I say, amazed that we're having this conversation at all. But glad actually.

'God, let's not get too wanky with each other or we'll lose

our competitive edge at work! Now, let's sit down cross-legged and discuss this ship thing or Miss will tell us off.'

Tara is a hoot! Her sense of humour doesn't come across at work at all. I think it's because we're surrounded by all these men with their own humour, one that's so different from our own. The other directors don't seem to get my sarcasm, like, it annoys them, as if they're left out of the joke and can't be in charge of it. Something like that. Some of the other managers and staff below me are deliciously sarcastic and we banter a bit at work now and again, but as I've said before, it goes nowhere in friendship terms because of my role. Nobody trusts HR.

'Tara, you're so different at work! Like a whole other person.'

'Well, you too! I mean, we all are, aren't we? Maybe we're different ships at work at home. See what I did there?'

We laugh. Then we talk about the ship thing. We talk about our lives outside of work, about our pasts, about the ships we used to be and the battles we've been through that have replaced all our planks. I tell her about my dad dying, my husband leaving, my mum and sis abroad.

'Most of the time I'm very content with my life choices. I wanted to focus on my career and stay here. I didn't want what my ex-husband wanted, so we mutually agreed to part. I like my own company. But I will admit that there are times when it strikes me how very solitary I am.'

I think back to that jibe Tara threw at me at work, about me being lonely. It was rotten to hear it at the time. But something about being in this room, about how Clio fosters being open and frank, encourages me to go further.

'And all right, I'll admit it. Like you said to me at work

that time: sometimes, I am lonely. Sometimes the loneliness gets to me.'

Tara looks down at her feet, then looks up at me.

'That was a shitty, cheap jibe and I'm sorry for it.'

Wow, I did not expect that.

'Thanks,' I say. Then I wonder something. 'Did people at work really gossip about me being lonely?'

'Nope,' says Tara, looking away, somewhat shamefaced. 'Derek made a passing reference to it once, in a jokey way.'

'What a dick,' I mutter.

'Well, yeah,' says Tara. 'It there's a consensus at work about anything, it's that Derek is most definitely a dick.'

That makes us both smile.

'Your turn now to spill the beans, Tara.'

What Tara tells me opens up a whole other side of her I had no idea about.

'You know what you were saying about loneliness,' Tara begins, 'well, I know exactly what you mean. Even though my situation is totally different from yours. You are alone at home and it gets to you sometimes. But you know what? There are times where I would kill to be in an empty house on my own. Bloody hell, I'd love it! I have two sons and a loving husband. Our kids are Josh who's seventeen and Manish who's fifteen. And my husband is Paranjay. We met at uni and married young. I kept my maiden name at work, Harryman. I've always kept work and home separate. I adore my kids, and my husband is a great husband. He works in IT and has put his career on hold, turning freelance so I can pursue mine more easily. That's why I've wanted this promotion so badly, to get to the top of my profession. To make all the sacrifice worth it. All the times I've let down the kids and

Paranjay. He's been great about it. The kids are great about it, which I know I should be grateful for. But sometimes I want to throw a hand grenade into my life so badly. I feel lonely in my own home sometimes, surrounded by people. I guess I've sacrificed a lot for my career. I've worked my backside off for years now and my husband has become the main caregiver at home. Which is fine. We both discussed it and it's what we agreed. But there is a price to pay. I sometimes feel like my kids don't really know me because I'm never there. Paranjay is pretty fed up with me much of the time because I don't listen to him properly. I know I don't and I try. But I've always got a million other things on my mind about work. I've missed out on most of the boys' key milestones and I feel constantly guilty about my kids and also my ageing parents who are in a home and I visit when I can. So, yeah, I'm literally surrounded by people at work and at home twenty-four-seven and all I want to do is run away and hide. I'd kill for a secret flat I could go to and just . . . be . . . alone. Alone with my thoughts. For five minutes. That's how I ended up doing this wellness stuff. It was an excuse to not be at home, or to be allowed to be in a room alone pretending to be really into yoga and not be asked for things and told things and badgered for things. And maybe wellness was an excuse also to just look for something else that was not work and not home, something *beyond*, something with some meaning. And meeting Clio. It's my one escape of the week and I'm desperately grateful for it. Thank God for Clio.'

Listening to Tara talk about her life, it's like watching that ship magically assemble from all the different parts, the old planks and the new planks coming together to build this interesting, complex and whole person. Wow, how I've

214

misjudged and misunderstood her. And how much we have in common despite our lives being so different. I feel the same as Tara about this promotion – a prize somehow for all the sacrifices I've chosen to make in my own life, to focus completely on my work to the detriment of every other aspect of my life, physically and mentally. I realise at this moment that meeting Clio and finding out that there is something beyond normal life, something extraordinary that happens in your mind when you open it up to possibility – I've been searching for something beyond too. Beyond work, for me. Work has been my whole life for so long, I truly had forgotten there was anything beyond it. Now I've tapped into these extraordinary visions Clio has gifted to me, I wonder what other possibilities there are in my mind, beyond my work brain. Something deeper, more fulfilling.

There's so much I want to say to Tara about what she's told me. But I can't frame it all. So I just reach over and give her a hug. She hugs me back. It's daft really. I don't even know why we're doing it. But as we pull back and look around us, loads of other women are giving each other hugs too. And at the front, on her podium, watching it all with a small, sweet smile is Clio. How wonderful it must be for her to see how well her work has turned out for everyone in the room, all discovering such important things about themselves and connecting with other women at the same time.

'Clio is amazing,' says Tara, reverently.

'Isn't she just,' I reply.

At that moment, Clio calls us all to go back to our mats to finish the session off. We do a couple of stretches sitting down, then place our palms together and everyone says 'Namaste' and then everyone claps and says, 'Thank you, Clio.' They must've done this before. Well, I know the drill now. Then Clio addresses us.

'Thank you for a wonderful session. Nothing I do has any meaning without you guys, every single one of you, remember that. One more thing before I let you go for lunch: thinking about our ship and the battles our ships have been through . . . as many of you know, I myself have battled cancer and survived.'

At this, there is a spontaneous and lengthy round of applause, as well as a couple of whoops from the audience. I join in, of course.

'In fact, it's my four-year cancer-versary this week, since I was first diagnosed and went very steeply into a sharp and sudden decline in health. My body was not my own. I was staring oblivion in its shadowy face. And this has brought about a moment of contemplation for me. To think how low I sank then, back in 2021. And to think how far I've come since. As many of you know as well, I rejected chemo and fought my own battle through my own nutrition programme, examples of which are on the app which all of you have now. Thank you for supporting the app. I know too that many of you have had personal experience of this terrible disease – either yourself or a close family member or friend. Everyone in this room has donated regularly to the cancer charities that I support by opting to include a payment when you book appointments with me. Thank you, from the depths of my soul, for this generosity that will help so many others in need. I want to congratulate you on your support for this and give you all a well-deserved round of applause.'

Everyone claps again and there are more whoops this time. I always donate each time I've booked with Clio. It feels good to know that while I can afford to get my own wellness help with Clio, at the same time I'm helping other people who really need it. Because this wellness business is expensive. It's only accessible to those who can afford it. So many people can't. And to help them in some small way through my donation, that's been my weekly dose of good vibes. We finish applauding and all look pleased with ourselves.

Clio continues: 'So I'm asking you today if you wish to keep helping others with cancer, that you go on a brand-new tab on my app that allows you to donate regularly by direct debit. There's an option to donate weekly, monthly, annually or as a one-off. This money will be used to help individuals with their cancer treatment and support. You'll see the names of the charities involved on the page: the Cancer Kids Amazing Treatment Fund and the Polly Twelvetrees Trust. Many of you are aware that I've been collecting for these charities for some time but I felt it would work even better if I put this option on the app and people could kindly agree to donate regularly. It's entirely up to you, of course, but please know that these charities do a magnificent job and deserve our help. Well, that's enough about that because I bet you're all ravenous for lunch so I'll shut up now!'

Everyone laughs and Clio says she'll see us all later for the afternoon session. Tara grabs her handbag from the side of the room. I really cannot wait to sit at lunch with Tara and talk more. I get the feeling she feels the same way but as soon as she pulls her phone from her bag, her face falls.

'Oh, for fuck's sake,' she says, bitterly.

'Everything okay?' I ask.

'Loads of messages from Paranjay. Some drama with Manish and his GCSE revision or something. He's had a meltdown. See what I mean? It never ends! Sorry, Lucy, I need to go and ring him.'

'No worries,' I say. 'I'll save you a seat at lunch. See you later.'

I wander out of the room slowly, thoughtfully. I glance over at Clio on her podium, seeing her chatting animatedly with a couple of the women. People are lingering, looking longingly at Clio. They don't want to leave the room. Everyone seems to want to go over there and talk to her. But many don't have the nerve to queue up. I feel the same way – I don't want this sensation to end, the atmosphere of this room and its mini loving democracy that will vaporise into thin air out in the real world. But I've no excuse to stay, so I meander over to the door. If only real life were like a class with Clio.

Lunch is in the same room as breakfast and it's a buffet again, but at least there are some carbs this time – broccoli and tomato quiche, bread and boiled potatoes – and I take a seat at one of the tables and look around to see if Tara is coming. Instead I catch the eye of Bitchy Sheridan – dressed head to toe in shades of pink activewear with hair newly curled and up in two bunches which make her look like a fifty-three-year-old seven-year-old – who waves manically at me with one hand while her other hand is carrying her plate. She hurries over and sits down next to me. Surely she has loads of other people here she'd rather sit with. Why does it have to be me, for fuck's sake?

'How's it all going with Clio Kenton then? Good stuff?' says Bitsy, picking at her plate full of food and hardly eating a thing. I'm meanwhile demolishing this quiche. Carbs and fat, at bloody last.

'Really well. She did an amazing session this morning. Totally blew my mind.'

'She is a wonder, isn't she?' says Bitchy, looking starry-eyed. 'I've based my career on her, you know. I mean my current career. I was an estate agent for years. I've only just started out as a yoga teacher and it's not going very well so far, to be horribly frank. But Clio gives me hope. She's gone through so much. And now look at her!'

'Well, yes, she's been through hell all right.'

'And been so brave. I've had conversations with her when she's been here dealing with stuff with Ma and Pop about the hall, you know. She's so inspirational when she talks about her cancer. You know she healed herself? Through nutrition alone. Isn't that incredible? She's basically cured her own cancer. And such a nasty cancer too.'

Bitchy spears a potato with her fork, looks at it and then pushes it off onto the plate again. God, it's so depressing watching her eat, or rather, not eat. It makes me wonder if she has some kind of issues with food. I don't. I'm still shovelling it in.

'Yes, my grandma had cervical cancer too, same as Clio,' I reply, trying to keep the conversation going, though I truly don't want to talk to Bitchy Sheridan about anything. As we talk, the table is filling up with other women and at this rate there won't be any room for Tara

'Bowel cancer, you mean,' says Bitchy.

'No, cervical,' I say.

'No,' replies Bitchy, pointedly. 'It was definitely bowel cancer. Clio told me all about it because my cousin Minty had bowel cancer and they treated her at the same hospital, the Royal Marsden in London.'

I have to take a mental leap over the fact that Bitchy's cousin is called Minty. Something to make Tara laugh later. But this sad news about Bitchy's cousin needs responding to.

'I'm sorry to hear that. How did it go for your cousin?'

'She's okay, thanks. She's had to change her diet completely, after the surgery. I'm doing my best to help her with a nutrition programme I've devised based on the stuff Clio has told me. It's not easy. The Royal Marsden were amazing though. Clio recommended it to me as the best place to go as they treated her so magnificently there.'

'Ah right,' I say, but then something jars. Royal Marsden? 'Your cousin wasn't at Maidstone Hospital then? I thought that's where Clio had gone.'

'No, the Royal Marsden. In London, of course. Nowhere round here would have a clue about proper treatment, for fudge's sake. As Clio said to me, it's all local yokels in the NHS round here. Deadly.'

'I must've got it wrong,' I say. But I'm thinking something quite different – Clio definitely said it was Maidstone Hospital that treated her. And she said she had cervical cancer, not bowel. Maybe she had both. That can happen, of course it does. That explains it. She had both. Even more awful for poor Clio.

I'm thinking about this and laying into the potatoes now which I've plastered with mayo, when Bitchy changes the subject abruptly.

'Listen, I'm so sorry but I must confess I don't remember knowing you at school. I feel terrible about it. But on this journey I'm on, with my yoga, and my wellness voyage, I've learnt that honesty is by far the best policy. I want to be truthful and honest with every human I meet. Could you tell me how we knew each other? Because I don't think we were in a badminton club together, were we? And can you remind me of your name? I'm so sorry.'

Bitchy looks so mortified by what she's said, I feel bad for her. And quite impressed that she has actually fessed up in such an honest and rather disarming manner.

'I'm Lucy,' I say.

'Lucy, it's lovely to meet you – again! I'm Bitsy!'

'Yeah, I know that,' I say and then I catch the honesty bug from Bitchy and decide to fess up myself. 'Okay, well, to be totally honest with you, Bitsy, we weren't friends. We didn't play badminton together. In the spirit of honesty, I want to tell you I was joshing you, teasing you. Messing you about. I'm sorry about that. But again, in the spirit of honesty, you know, Bitsy, you were really quite horrible to me at school. I know you don't remember me but I was the one who you called Doughnut Dinah. Does that ring a bell?'

Bitsy's face is blank, then literally colours red as she drops her head. I don't say a thing. I savour the moment and chew on a big bite of baguette slathered in butter. I feel curiously at peace having told her that. An exorcism from my past.

Then Bitchy speaks. 'I wish I could say I don't remember that, that I'd never say something like that. But I did say that. It was me. And I'm sorry. I'm really sorry . . . for being such a bitch.'

Wow. Okay. That's pretty full on. And again, honest. And I have to respect that.

'Well, my mate Jac and I used to call you Bitchy. And I still do call you Bitchy in my head.'

She nods and just accepts it, takes the blow.

'I don't blame you,' she replies. 'I *was* a bitch back then.

But I hope you can see the journey I've been on. I think my cousin's cancer had a part to play in that. It humbled me, helping her through that. We were raised together. My mum's sister moved in with us for a while and my cousin and I became like sisters. When she was ill, I heard all this language about fighting back against cancer and all I could think of was, why does it have to be a battle? If you lose, and the worst happens – that you actually die – does that mean you're weak and a loser? That seemed the most unfair thing to say to a person with a disease. So yeah, it humbled me. I promise you I'm not the person I was. And I'm sorry I said those shitty things. I can only imagine how hard that was for you and I'm really bloody sorry.'

Gosh, this really is a weekend for revelations. Suddenly, Bitchy Sheridan has become a whole person. The whole damn ship is sitting there before me of the real Bitsy.

'Thank you,' I say, simply.

'And,' she says, giving me a cheery look up and down, 'you look just great now! That's why I didn't recognise you, I bet! You're looking . . . ' She's searching around for a suitable hyperbole that I won't believe. 'Just fabulous these days, Lucy!'

'Thanks again.'

'You're welcome,' says Bitsy, simply. Somehow, I don't want to call her Bitchy anymore.

There's lots I could say to her but I don't. Something about Bitsy's vulnerability has mended that hole in my soul that the bullying tore all those years ago. It's pretty incredible to feel that hole just gone now. So I put my arm around Bitsy's shoulders and give her a little hug and she makes a small sound of surprise, but then relaxes into it. It's good for both of us, I know, in that moment.

I've finished my lunch, so I stand up, smile down at Bitsy and walk away. I may have bonded with my old bully but that doesn't mean I want to sit and be best friends with her. She's still an annoying person, despite her honesty. But it has done me good to hear that from her. Yes, she was a bitch at school. But what's the point of retaining that kind of hate for her all these years later? People do dumb, careless things when they're teenagers. I remember laughing when a girl in my class told me her grandad was killed by a pigeon. I mean, it sounds funny! I never found out how the pigeon killed him because I laughed so much she wouldn't tell me. Did the pigeon fly into his face when he was on his bicycle? Who knows. But anyway, yes, teenagers can be pretty awful human beings sometimes but can grow into perfectly good people. Maybe that's what's happened with Bitsy. All right, she's pretentious. But she's also been perfectly friendly to me now. Maybe it's another lesson here, to get rid of old woes and start afresh. As Clio said, none of us are the same ship we used to be. I want to be that new ship.

Chapter 20

I go back to my room and wash my face and clean my teeth, ready for the afternoon session. I won't recount the whole thing here, because it's a similar mix of physical and mental stuff, some things about accepting the person you are now and living in the present. Plus more yoga stuff this time and a session of meditation, which doesn't work for me at all, as I literally cannot turn off my inner voice. But I'm not focusing on it fully, because there is one thing that's bothering me and that's the fact that Tara isn't here. She didn't come to lunch and she isn't at the afternoon session. I hope she's okay. We have a work group WhatsApp for the directors and she's in there, but I've never messaged her individually. I wonder if I should when the session ends.

When I'm back in my room, sitting on my bed, having changed clothes for dinner, I message Tara individually, asking if she's okay. No reply for now. I had to set up a new WhatsApp message page for her – does she get the message if I'm not saved on her phone? I've no idea. God, I'm so bad with tech. While I'm waiting for dinner to start, I go on Clio's app and find the extra cancer charities page. I have a look at their home pages and they do great work for folk with cancer, funding research, helping people with alternative treatments and taking kids with terminal cancer on cool days out. I sign up on Clio's app straight away, paying £15 a month for each charity. That's not much, I know, but all this wellness stuff has cost me a fortune and I'm going to have to take it easy on spending for a while. I do have savings but I've generally always treated those as sacrosanct, in case of emergency, and the bulk of my savings are not readily accessible, to make it less likely I'll dip into them for trivial purposes. When you're self-sufficient with nobody on this earth to rely on, you have to make sure you're protected from disaster, if you can afford to, of course, which not everybody can. Luckily for me, my wage allows me to do that and I am very careful with my money. It's a responsibility that comes from living alone. You know, I hate that word 'alone'. It rarely comes with a positive spin. It sounds too much like loneliness, which is a whole other thing. I've googled it before – how to term living alone in a more positive way – and all I could come up was solitudinarian (someone who lives a secluded lifestyle) or anchoress (feminine version of anchorite = a kind of hermit). But I'm not a hermit, not some kind of monk who needs to live an ascetic lifestyle. Other words that pop up are unmarried, unattached, spouseless. All those uns and lesses label you as lacking something that you should have. Makes me mad. I *choose* to live the way I live. There should be a better word for people like me. How about spousefree? Or even better, no mention of spouse at all, for even that suggests that it should be part of everyone's 'normal' situation. Fuck that. I'm going to make a neologism for people like me, living alone by choice and loving it, and that is self-homer. I'll copyright that! (Can you copyright a word? Probably Tara will know. She's our legal adviser, after all.) Yeah, that's me. I'm a self-homer and proud.

It's time for dinner. I decide I can get an early night after that and have a bath and pack. Tonight it's another buffet and this time it's loads of meat and fish and roasted veg, so something for the carnivores at last. I end up next to two women while we're dishing out our food. They're a bit older than me. They're in another group of Clio's and are doing a bunch of other classes this weekend. There are plenty of other classes that I could choose from to go to today, all included in the price, but – I don't know – they all sound annoying to me. The kind of stuff I had in the January Rejuvenate, way-out, wacky stuff based on energy and so forth. Still not a fan. Plus I won't be going to Bitsy's yoga sessions, thanks, however reformed she is. So, I know I'm not really getting value for money this weekend, but I'm getting what I need and that is time away from time, a hiatus from my very bloody stressful life and an opportunity to see more of Clio. Plus, a useful by-product, getting to know Tara, though she still isn't here and no message. Has she gone home? Anyway, I start talking to these other two women instead, forcing myself to be sociable, for once. They're chatty and nice enough and not wearing designer activewear, which is a bonus. Both in relaxed jersey trousers and sweatshirts. They seem a bit more normal to normal old me. I'm feeling braver after having been here a day now. They're both in their early sixties, I'm guessing – sixty-four or thereabouts. As we put our plates down on a table, one of the women mouths that she's going to the loo and nips out.

I carry on chatting with the other woman about the day's events and what we've learnt about ourselves. And then, inevitably, the topic of conversation turns to how wonderful Clio is.

'She really is, isn't she?' I say.

'Truly,' she says. 'She got me through so many bad times in my life.'

'I'm sorry to hear that. But glad too that Clio helped you.'

'Oh, she saved my life, no doubt. I had a terrible relationship with my mother and brother and so did Clio, exactly the same, a toxic, poisonous relationship with both, especially her brother. I had cut them out of my life completely and felt terribly guilty about it.'

I remember what Clio said about cutting her family out of her life too. I thought she said a sister but it must've been brother. My post-menopause memory is terrible.

The woman carries on, 'But then Clio helped me see that removing people from your life is just as necessary as removing black mould from your bathroom wall, you know? Just knowing that she was able to leave her family behind and still make it to where she is today. My brother made my life hell for years and so did Clio's, until she put her foot down five years ago and left her family behind and never looked back. That changed everything for me.'

Now I'm confused. Clio left home at sixteen, didn't she? Or is it my crap memory again? It's so frustrating not being able to rely on your own memory. I ask the lady just in case.

'I thought Clio had a sister and hadn't seen her family since she was a teenager.'

The woman shakes her head emphatically. 'No, not at all. She has a brother and stopped seeing him and her mother just before Covid hit. The lockdown changed everything for her. Has she not told you about that?'

'No . . . ' I say, and think back to the conversation with Clio about our families. I must've misunderstood. 'Well,' I add brightly, 'I'm really glad she was able to help you with that.'

'Oh, she has. But not only me. Ah, here's my friend. Her life has literally been saved by Clio! She'll tell you all about it, I'm sure. She does talks about it at the WI and other places. She wants to spread the word about how Clio has helped her.'

The lady's friend comes back and sits down. They introduce themselves. The woman I've been speaking to with the horrid brother is Imelda and her friend is Caroline. They both have the exact same haircut – pure white, short at the back and spiky on top, like a uniform. I wonder if I'll automatically chop my hair off the moment I turn sixty. Lots of older women here have that cut.

'Imelda tells me that Clio saved your life, literally,' I say to Caroline. 'And that you give talks about it?'

Caroline, who is wearing big round glasses that make her look like a benevolent owl, replies, 'Yes, well, cancer isn't easy for anyone, of course. I lost my husband to it.'

'Oh God, I'm so sorry to hear that. I lost my dad to cancer too. Seven years ago.'

'I'm sorry for your loss. It was three years ago now for me. My husband was the love of my life. It doesn't get easier. It just changes. Over time. Last year, I made plans to end it all. Literally. I was going to end my life. I had plans on how to do it. Then a friend suggested Clio. She was a shining light in a dark tunnel for me. She talked me through the pain. She had the same cancer as my husband, you see. She knew what my husband had gone through with his thyroid cancer. Except it's usually one that can be treated quite successfully. But my husband went into respiratory failure. And we sadly lost him. Thank heavens Clio's thyroid cancer was able to be treated.'

'Thyroid cancer?' I repeated.

'Yes, as I say, it's usually quite treatable. My husband was the unlucky one. Clio told me all of the measures she took to avoid chemo and radiotherapy and how it worked to reduce her thyroid cancer to the point of remission and where she needed no more treatment. I give talks about that now, about Clio's teachings and her advice about how to beat cancer the natural way. It's life-changing.'

There's that word again, life-changing. Tara used it. I've used it. Everyone says that about Clio.

At that moment, someone taps me on the shoulder. It's Tara – at last.

'Are you okay?' I say straight away, because she does not look okay. She looks hassled and frazzled and severely fed up.

'Not really. I've been back and forth home to sort out this domestic drama. Manish is having a meltdown about his exams. He flunked his mocks and he thinks he's a loser. It's all going to shit.'

'Oh Christ, that sounds heavy. Come and get some dinner. It's real, actual *food* food today.'

Tara swiftly shakes her head.

'I can't, I'm sorry. I'm just back to pack up my stuff and then I'll be off.'

'But you'll miss your one-to-one with Clio! Don't go. Let your husband deal with it.'

'I can't. I wish I could. But I'm needed. Look, I'll see you at work on Monday. I'm really, really glad we did this.' Tara nods at me and smiles, though grimly.

'Me too,' I say. 'Take care.'

'See you soon,' she says and rushes off out of the dining room.

I really feel for Tara at that moment. This was *her* time, something away from work and home and all that responsibility. It really sucks that she's had to miss most of it. Plus I was looking forward to having more chats, to be honest. Whatever happens with the promotion, I'm actually really glad I have another woman at the top level at work I can talk to.

By the time I've had that conversation, Imelda and Caroline are animatedly talking to two other women on the same table and I'm suddenly very tired. I get up and thank Imelda for the chat.

After my bath and ensconced on the bed in a hotel towelling robe, I think about Tara's busy life and it reminds me of my sister Shirl. With her kids and husband and Mum to look after, I bet her daily schedule resembles something similar to Tara's, or at least Tara's husband's. I'm run off my feet enough with work alone. I literally can't fathom how people do all of that with families as well. I decide to message Shirl. I've actually been messaging her weekly recently. Things are better than they were. I tell her a bit about this wellness weekend and the cool new things I'm learning about myself.

Then I add:

I know that might sound a bit self-indulgent. I know you don't have much time for anything like that in your busy

life. But I would urge you to carve out time for yourself, Shirl. You need to prioritise yourself sometimes too.

I see the bobble head pop up that shows Shirl has seen my messages.

She replies:

I don't have time to breathe! But I'm glad you do!

Then she adds,

That sounded bitter. But actually I am glad. I feel like you've changed recently. Mum is really happy you're in touch more. It means a lot to her, you know. I don't want to fall out with you. I know you give a damn, not much of a damn, but a bit of a damn, at least.

I'd say I give at least 83% of a damn.

You're massaging the stats there, sis. Typical businesswoman.

All right, fair enough. Look, I've got to go now and get some sleep as it's my last day of wellness tomorrow. Sending love.

Xx

Just as I'm finishing off with Shirl, I get a text from Jacqui, just saying,

Hey

Hey!

I'm sorry, about all the shit.

Me too.

We don't need to say any more. We've had little spats before, though this one felt worse. But we know we love each other. We don't need a big heart to heart to mend it all. Nothing's been broken.

I think it's hilarious you've just seen Bitchy. I'd totally forgotten about that wingnut.

I want to tell her about how Bitsy's a reformed character (mostly). But somehow I feel like Jacqui won't understand. She'll still want to laugh at Bitsy and she'll think I'm being holier than thou. Despite the fact that Jacqui and I have made up, I still feel like I'm a long way from her now, not just because I'm away from home, but because this journey I'm on has somehow moved me away from our friendship a bit.

But then, Jacqui texts,

Sorry about saying fuck you.

It doesn't matter. It's fine. I love you.

I love you too, you idiot. See you soon? How about next Saturday?

Yes, I can do that. Looking forward to it xx

232

Despite her apology, those messages leave me feeling at odds with her. I know we tease each other but – I don't know – I felt a little jolt when she called me an idiot. Am I overreacting? Probably. But I call myself an idiot often enough not to want to hear it from my best friend too. Plus I really don't know how to explain to her how life-changing this weekend with Clio has been.

Then I think about Clio. She's been a revelation. But then . . . I have a little niggle. This business of Clio's cancer. Clio told me she had cervical cancer. And she told Bitsy she had bowel cancer. And now she's told this woman Caroline that she had thyroid cancer. I mean, could it have metastasised so far? Maybe it could, cancer travels around the body, everybody knows that. I google it. It is possible to have cervical, bowel and thyroid cancer but it is very rare. Well, she's a rare person, is Clio. Maybe she had that rare cancer. Well, she must've done and that's that.

But what about the stuff that Imelda said about Clio's family? A brother and mother who she cut off in 2020? Clio said she cut them out at sixteen. Maybe she got back in touch with them. Maybe she had both a sister and a brother and didn't mention him. I mean, the truth is, I know so little about her. Clio has told me little snippets about her life and I'm trying to make a thousand-piece jigsaw out of a handful of pieces. And Imelda and Caroline have clearly known Clio a lot longer than me. It's silly of me to think I know her because of tiny crumbs of information she's given me in the few weeks I've been aware of her existence. I really need to stop inventing problems in my head. I am so prone to that. I make a pact with myself that I'm not allowed to overthink or catastrophise for one week from today. Good, that's that sorted, then.

And with that, I actually get a very good night's sleep. Roseland Hall's beds are heavenly.

* * *

Sunday comes and it's time for my long-awaited one-to-one with Clio, just half an hour, so she can fit everyone in. She arranges to meet me in my room, making it easier to move between clients. She starts by pulling out a tote bag with Clarity with Clio emblazoned across the front in swirly writing. I assume I'm going to be given some kind of free goodie-bag – which would be welcome considering the vast cost of this weekend – and I get a little giddy, like a kid in the queue at the end of a birthday party waiting for their cake slice wrapped in a napkin and their little bag of favours. But it turns out the bag is not for me. Instead, Clio pulls out what she tells me is 'a handpicked selection of products from the stalls that I have an inkling you might be interested in'. She shows me each one and I'm obliged to hold them and look. There are personalised vitamins – each with a sticker with my name printed on it – plus a selection of tubs of sleep drink powders and bottles of shower products. Clio is really singing their praises and I'm starting to feel a bit pushed into buying them, but I don't. I've spent quite enough this weekend.

'I'll have a think about it,' I say, smiling, being polite, but actually I'm a little annoyed about it. I have to remind myself, though, that Clio is an independent businesswoman and has to make a living. And it was nice to see that the vitamins had been picked out exclusively for me. (Or maybe they just stick a sticker on the same pot for everyone . . .)

'Of course,' says Clio and smiles broadly at me. 'I'll send you the links by email so you can look into them more.'

'Thanks,' I say. I would really rather get on with the session now, because we've already lost ten minutes of thirty to this stuff.

'Okay, so, moving on,' says Clio, ever the mind-reader. 'What do you feel you've learnt this weekend?'

'Well, I loved the ship story. And yoga. I managed to settle an old score which was actually healing. Also I made a new friend.'

'Tara,' says Clio, definitively.

'Yes. We were work rivals. Well, we still are. We're both up for the same promotion when the old CEO leaves in a few weeks. But we've managed to get past that. And now we've got a bit of a friendship starting, I think. I never expected that in a million years.'

'I just knew you two would hit it off,' says Clio, blue eyes sparkling. 'That's just what I wanted.'

I can see she's orchestrated this and actually I'm grateful.

Clio adds, 'And I'm so thrilled that you've found this weekend useful and it will help you to move on with your work and family issues and most importantly your grief for your father's death. I do think that's at the bottom of a lot of these issues, Lu. Cancer is a thief that robs us of our loved ones and turns our own bodies against us. But we can take grief and we can take cancer and we can change it and fight it and beat it. Believe me, I know.'

And now we're back to cancer. At her mention of it, those niggling doubts from last night swell again in my overthinking brain. Why did Clio not tell me she had three types of cancer?

Then, I can't help myself. Call it my habit of extracting

salient information from people at work as director of HR, trying to get the actual truth from differing workers about what really happened. I have to be able to see through the defensiveness and bullshit that people talk when they're cornered. It must be that instinct because, without even really wanting to, I feel compelled to ask Clio more about this cancer issue. But I can't just come out with it. I'll have to find a more roundabout way of saying it.

'Clio, I just wanted to say how sorry I am that you've had more than one type of cancer. I can't even fathom how difficult it must have been for you.'

'Yes,' says Clio, steadily. She looks curiously at me. Actually, she looks a bit uncomfortable. Something tells me to push her to talk about it, even though all my normal rules of conversation would say that this is wrong, that it's being too nosy and disrespectful. But Clio means so much to me now, that this niggling doubt I have in my head has to be silenced.

'I was talking yesterday to an old school acquaintance, Bitsy – her parents own Roseland Hall.'

'Of course, I know Bitsy via her parents. Lovely people.'

'Yes . . . ' I say and pause. 'Well, I was talking to Bitsy and she told me about her cousin's bowel cancer and how you had that too. And then I spoke to a lady called Caroline and she told me about your thyroid cancer too. It must've been so hard travelling between different hospitals to get the right treatment. And to have such a rare situation of it metastasising to the thyroid. It makes me respect you all the more, for everything you've been through. I'm just so happy you're well now.'

'Thank you,' says Clio and she smiles but it's an odd smile, as if there is no life behind it. Am I imagining that? Something tells me I need to push on. I need to get to the bottom of this. It's too important not to.

'And I was talking to Imelda too and she told me about how you had your family back in your life again – after you left at sixteen – and then you cut them out again in 2020, including a brother. It sounds like your family life has been pretty harrowing. I'm so sorry you've had to go through all of that, Clio.'

There is a distinct pause while Clio looks away, down at her feet. Then she looks up. Her face looks . . . different somehow. Like a mask.

'I don't really talk about it. I don't like to talk about any of it, Lucy. My cancer. My family. It is private.'

I feel chastised. And I note that she called me Lucy, not Lu. I feel told off and put in my place. But I also feel I was out of order. I mean, what if it's all just something I've concocted in my mind?

'Of course it is,' I say. 'I'm sorry. The last thing I would ever want is to intrude.'

I feel like she's turned from hot water to cold at the flick of a switch. Oh God, why did I start talking about this anyway? It was a stupid, crass thing to do. I try to save the situation. 'I was just . . . so moved by what I heard from your different clients about your life. It was . . . inspirational.'

'Thank you. But just a reminder that we have a therapist to client relationship and my whole life is not open to my clients. A certain . . . distance must be maintained.'

Now I feel the frost settling over me. Have I blown it with Clio? Oh God, please not that. I need her.

'Of course. I'm sorry. Please accept my apologies. I am so sorry.'

'Don't be. But listen, you are here for you, to talk about you. So let's focus on you, shall we, Lu?'

She's calling me Lu again. That's a relief. Clio smiles at me just as brightly and bids me goodbye just as kindly. So maybe I haven't messed it up with Clio. She seems back to her normal, warm self again and I leave relieved that I haven't blown the best thing that's happened to me since the invention of the KitKat Chunky.

I don't stay for lunch, as I can't bear another buffet and neither can my bowels. They need a square meal of one thing. I stop and get a Sizzler from KFC drive-thru on the way home. It's horrible and wonderful all at once. My latest healthy eating kick lasted two days then. But I'm not worried about that. I had a phenomenal time in Clio's classes. And I've been taken utterly by surprise by Tara's revelations.

It has been an incredible weekend, I think.

Mostly.

Chapter 21

It's Sunday evening and I'm in bed, phone in hand, ready to book in my next session with Clio. It's strange but I miss having her around. It was such a comforting feeling staying at Roseland Hall and knowing she was there in the same building. I think a lot of her clients must've felt like that. I'm also a bit worried about the way our session went this morning and that she's a bit annoyed with me. I hope not. She was certainly perfectly nice when our session ended. So, I'm on her site and booking in – I do hope next Friday is still free. I click to book and the screen just goes blank. I try again. Several times. I click out of the page and reload it. But the same thing happens. Oh well, there must be a glitch on the site. I'll email her instead. So I do and tell her I couldn't book on the site and would like to do it by email instead, please, for Friday night. And I tell her how wonderful the weekend was. That should sort it.

* * *

Back at work, it's so nice to actually get on with Tara, at last. We are a bit awkward with each other at first, as if we've been to Fight Club and nobody talks about Fight Club. But we ease into it and we're easier with each other as the week goes on. I ask her about the GCSE drama with her son and she says it's passed now. Parenthood is just a series of narrowly missed disasters, she tells me. I've certainly got that impression from Jacqui and Shirl's lives as mothers. Constant firefighting. I've not had to have that many dealings with Tara in my average work week – I spend most of my time chastising middle managers and their staff about their ridiculous behaviour. This week a junior employee in Risk decided to wear a T-shirt that reads: *I'm no gynaecologist but I know a cunt when I see one*. Well, I can't say I disagree. But it's not exactly appropriate workwear, so we have that ridiculous argument and the idiot threatens to take her T-shirt off and wear her bra only at work all day. We narrowly avoid that. Another day, another pointless spat. Oh, to be COO . . . The conference and the prospect of promotion is looming in around four weeks, that's all. And despite Tara and I being the prime rivals for this post, when I have seen Tara this week, we get on really well. There's a kind of unwritten rule that we don't discuss the promotion. What will be will be, may the best woman win, and all that. It's just nice to have a friend at work, a woman at the same level as me, after all these years of female isolation. It's just the tonic I need in my job.

By Thursday, I still haven't had a reply from Clio. What's going on? I won't get an appointment tomorrow by now, I shouldn't think. But I email again on Thursday night, just in case. Still nothing. Friday comes and goes and I spend the evening alone, worrying. At least I'm seeing Jacqui tomorrow for dinner. But I'm a bit worried about that too. I hope we can smooth things over.

We meet in a tapas restaurant that serves nice cocktails and I get a taxi so I can relax. The food is overpriced and nothing like the real tapas you get when you wander from bar to bar in Barcelona, or other Spanish places I've been on my delicious single holidays (I bloody love travelling alone. Nobody else's agenda to deal with). Jac comes in, resplendent in bootcut jeans and a shirt covered in bright green drawings of apples. She's a knockout, she really is. We hug and – hopefully – make up. I'm so relieved we can get back to normal.

Once we're sitting down and starting on our first cocktail, I apologise to her.

'What I said to you wasn't even true. I don't think you think I should stay the way I am. I don't think you think I'm a lonely thing who sits around waiting for you to need me. I don't even know where that came from. I was just being defensive and I'm really sorry.'

Jacqui reaches over and squeezes my arm.

'Don't worry about any of that. I know you didn't mean it. But sorry, chick. I'm not going to back down about Clio. I'm really worried about it.'

My hackles rise again but I'm determined not to fall out about it this time.

'I'm not sure it's a good idea to discuss Clio then,' I hedge and take a glug of my cocktail. I just want to have a nice time tonight.

But Jacqui wants to plough onwards. 'Look, you know I'm the one person in your life who will never, ever bullshit you. I will always tell you the truth and the facts. It's the journalist in me. Plus it's age. Now I'm in my fifties, I can't be arsed with constantly analysing people's feelings about hard truths. If someone is being a dick, then I'll tell them. You know that about me. And I am really worried that this Clio woman is doing a number on you. That she's going to try and turn you into one of these evangelical wellness nutters. And . . . well . . . '

Jacqui takes a deep draught of her potent cocktail, then shakes her head and closes her eyes.

She recovers and goes on, 'I'm worried I'm going to lose the sarcastic, kickass bitch who's my best friend.'

'That'll never happen,' I say and reach over and grab her hand. I'm a bit tipsy already as I haven't eaten much today and the tapas haven't arrived yet. I suddenly feel a bit emotional.

Jacqui goes on, 'There's nothing wrong with evolving as a person. I just want you to remember that having a healthy scepticism for things is good.'

'It's all right. I agree,' I say. 'I just want to be honest with you and have your support, that I've found this amazing new thing that is making me happy for the first time in ages.'

'I get that. And you know I love you and want that for you. I'm sorry I said fuck you.'

'No, don't be. I said some shitty things too. I'm sorry too.'

'Okay, we're all square then,' says Jacqui, but she doesn't look happy about it. Then she visibly tries to put on an amenable face. 'Tell me about this retreat then. I'll be more open-minded this time, I promise.'

At last, the little plates of tapas come and we start noshing, comparing patatas bravas and overcooked calamari. It's like old times. I've missed Jacqui this week. And the truth is, I really, really want to run something by her, something that's been bugging me all week.

'So, the weekend retreat was amazing. But there was something else . . .'

'What?'

'Well, I'll tell you the amazing bits first. The maddest thing was Bitsy Sheridan turning out not to be such a bitch after all. And even Tara too!'

'Was Tara there?'

I'd forgotten I hadn't told Jacqui that.

'God yeah! But it was fine. More than fine. Let me start at the beginning. There's so much to tell.'

'I'm all ears!'

I tell her all the ins and outs of the weekend and we have a riot laughing about Bitsy. Plus, Jacqui really does listen about the other stuff, the good stuff, the stuff that's changed me and helped me.

'I can see it means a lot to you. And I can see it might be good for you. In moderation. I'm still a bit worried about this Clio woman though, Lu. I had a quick look at her website tonight before I met you. Did you see she's not on any social media, not one platform? That just seems dodgy to me. In my experience, these days, the only people with businesses that need promoting – and yet who are ghosts on social media – are the ones with something to hide.'

Then, I order another pair of cocktails, because this bit needs lubrication. I know I've been defensive about Clio but the truth is, I'm having doubts. And I need to share them with the one person whose judgement I trust more than anyone.

243

'Listen, Jac. It's not the only thing that seems odd. I've spoken to a few people now about Clio. And every one of them has a different version of her story. According to each person, she's had several different cancers. And either has a brother or a sister or both and there's other stuff. It's just . . . a bit weird.'

I tell her all the details, about what Bitsy said, and Imelda and Caroline. And, as I guessed it might, Jacqui's face transforms from my friend into a bloodhound. She's sniffed out something all right. That's what her expression is telling me.

'What . . . the . . . fuck?!'

'I mean, it could all be explained away, right? Cancer spreads to different body parts. She could've just told different snippets of her past and they've mixed up in the retelling. I've got no proof whatsoever. But . . . I don't know . . . I'm starting to feel odd about it.'

Jacqui plonks her drink down on the bar and grabs my hands. We're both a bit pissed now.

'Okay . . . I'm going to hold back. For you, my friend. Because I know you'll shut up shop if I tell you what I'm really thinking. But look. If there is something dodgy about Clio – and I'm starting to get the distinct impression there might well be – then this isn't just about your private life. Clio's now in your work life too. You've arranged for her to do the keynote speech at your work conference.'

Oh God, I hadn't even thought about that. How could I have forgotten!

'Oh Christ,' I say and stare disaster in the face, if my worries about Clio's validity end up holding water.

'Can you cancel it, her speech?'

'God no, she's signed a contract. It's a done deal. Oh fffffuck.'

The alcohol makes everything feel worse, of course. My head is swimming with the implications of having recommended someone not wholly trustworthy to represent my own bid for promotion at the conference, about which I can see now I showed no due diligence. How could I have been so stupid? But then again, it's just suspicions at this point. I have no evidence either way. What if there is nothing dodgy going on? What if it's all a misunderstanding? And how can I find out? My mind is spiralling in a vortex of panic, off up into the sky like Dorothy's house in the tornado.

'Don't panic yet,' says Jacqui, bringing me back down to earth. 'Meet up with her. This needs sorting. You don't want her messing up for you at work. You need to talk to her about her presentation – use that as a pretext. I mean, it's not a pretext really. You ought to be checking out what she's actually going to be presenting. Your promotion is riding on this staff conference. Go and see her. Get it sorted.'

'I will, I will . . . But . . . but she's not answering my emails. I've sent her two this week after I couldn't book on her website.'

Jacqui grimaces and my heart sinks. Maybe it wasn't a coincidence that there was a so-called glitch on Clio's website. Maybe she blocked me from booking somehow. And now she's not answering my emails either.

'That's not a good sign. Get your phone out. Let's have another go on the site. I'll have a go too, see if it's just you.'

We both get our phones out. But before we have a chance to go on Clio's site, I see a notification that I have an email – from Clio!

'Read it out!' cries Jacqui.

> *Dear Lucy,*
> *So sorry for delay in replying. Bit of a crisis going on here. Just to say, apologies you couldn't book a session. I meant to explain this but this ongoing crisis has taken up all my brain space. Basically, since I've signed the contract to appear at your conference, I have a rule that I don't work with clients personally who I also work with professionally. I should've said that at the time but with everything going on I forgot. Please accept my apologies. I shall be seeing you in a few weeks at the end of March for the conference and I'm really looking forward to it.*
> *See you then and very best regards,*
> *Clio Kenton*
> *Therapeutic therapist and inspirational speaker*

'Therapeutic therapist,' says Jacqui, with a look of disgust.

'What do you think?' I say urgently. Could this be all it is? Just a simple explanation.

Jacqui hunches her shoulders. 'Could well be legit. Sounds legit . . . sort of.'

'What? Why sort of?'

'I dunno, darling. I just . . . my spidey senses are tingling.'

Jacqui is well known for her great instincts. She's just one of those people who can read other people and situations quickly and effectively. It's one of the things we've always bonded on, that we can see through bullshit. I need it in my job. I use it all the time. So how could I have let myself become hoodwinked in my private life?

'What about?'

'Well, first off, it's damn bloody convenient that she's made this decision about not seeing you as a client again *after* you spent a small fortune on her hugely overpriced weekend retreat.'

'Oh God, yeah. That's true.'

'Plus . . . there's something a lot worse that I reckon she's up to, Lu . . . '

I feel a bit sick now. Maybe it's just the cocktails. Maybe not.

'Like what? What do you mean? What is it we're actually saying about Clio here?'

There it is, the question of the night. And I don't want to hear the answer, I really don't.

'Honey, I want you to consider the very real possibility . . . that Clio . . . never . . . had . . . cancer . . . at all.'

That's a bombshell. What? How can . . . who would do that?

'Surely not! Who would lie about having cancer? That's disgusting.'

'Oh my God, haven't you heard of these social media influencers who've pretended to have cancer and got shitloads of money for it?'

'No??'

'Where have you been, under a *rock*? Too busy with work, that's your problem. Not enough time wasted on Instagram.'

'Christ, that is the lowest of the low, lying about cancer.'

'Right? Google it. There's been a few. Taken money for charities and not paid it. At least one's in prison now. Fucking awful.'

'At least they're in prison.'

'Not all of them. Plenty get away with it and just walk scot-free.'

'I can't . . . I can't believe it of Clio though. She's such a good person.'

But really, what proof do I have of that? Did she just seem to be a good person? I was paying her after all. Have I been so easily led down the garden path – me, with all my healthy scepticism and life experience?

'Look,' says Jacqui and forces my attention back to her as my thoughts spiral again. I feel like Jacqui is holding onto me while I fear being swept away. 'Maybe Clio is legit. Maybe none of this is dodgy. But I think you have to consider the possibility that she never had cancer at all. Maybe she just uses it as a grift to get people's sympathy. It might not be about the money. But either way, it sure is a convenient coincidence that you've not been able to see or book with Clio since you asked her about the cancer and her family.'

Then I realise that my secret fear is not that Clio is a con artist, but that I alienated her, by being too needy and getting obsessed with her. This makes me feel nauseous. How embarrassing.

'Maybe I blew it. Maybe Clio thought I was some uber-fan nutter who wanted access to all the most personal parts of her life. And she shut me out. My God, how humiliating.'

I feel so low. So small and ridiculous.

'No, no,' says Jacqui. 'Don't blame yourself! That's what she wants. You said those other women at the retreat – and Bitsy – they all talked about how Clio had shared personal stuff with them, so it wasn't that she didn't share anything with her clients, clearly. Think about all the holes in her story.'

'But we don't know that they are holes yet. It might just be that nobody has been given the whole story.'

Jacqui looks unconvinced. But then she shrugs and says, 'Yeah, it's possible. It's perfectly possible that nothing is really wrong. But just in case, since it's all wrapped up with work and the promotion now, you do need to have it out with her. Reply to her now and ask for the meeting. Get it done and you'll feel better.'

That's a great idea. I tap it out as Jacqui goes to order more food. These tiny plates of overpriced tapas are pointless for staving off the effects of cocktails. We definitely need more carbs. I tap out the email on my phone and show it to Jacqui when she gets back. I know we're both a bit drunk but I'm hoping that between us we're not too far gone to proofread an email. Basically, I just ask Clio for a meeting about the conference soon, so we can discuss her keynote speech. It's professional, friendly to a point, yet brief. Good. Sent.

'I've had another idea,' says Jacqui. 'Why not talk to someone else who's had meetings with Clio, before you meet with her about it? Get a bit more background info?'

'Well, yeah, that is a good idea. But who? I don't have any contact details with that whats-their-name at the thing – Imelda . . . Caroline. And I can't bear the idea of talking to Bitsy. But even if I did, I'm not sure she's reliable. I mean, we were mortal enemies once. The only other person is Tara, of course.'

'Talk to Tara, then.'

'But until very recently, we were enemies too. And we're still up against each other for this promotion. What if I share with Tara that I think Clio might be a grifter, then what happens about the staff conference? Getting Clio as a speaker was my big coup and if I've fucked that up, it will only benefit Tara.'

Jacqui grimaces again. Jacqui is always so positive with me, that when she makes that face, I know things are bad.

'Honestly, I don't think you have much choice. We'll just have to hope that Tara is a good enough person to not take advantage of that. You've talked to her. What do you think?'

I think about the way she was in the office, when she showed a pretty nasty streak about the promotion. Then I think how vulnerable she was in Clio's session at the retreat, baring her soul to me. Talk about opposites.

'I think . . . she's complicated. Like we all are.'

'Never a truer word spoken. Okay, well, message her tomorrow and ask for a meeting with her on Monday. That'll sort that. You can relax a bit then. You'll be well on the way to solving this, you'll see.'

Jacqui's planning and sensible words make me feel a bit more grounded.

'You're my anchor,' I say to Jacqui.

'I know. And you're mine. Everything is such a fucking mess right now.'

More food comes and we spend the next hour or so talking about her family issues, mostly about Harvey, her eldest, how he's still struggling with muscle weakness, which makes no sense for a strapping fifteen-year-old lad like him.

'We've got another GP appointment in three weeks but it feels like an age to wait.'

'I'm so sorry, my darling Jac. What can I do? Tell me what I can do.'

Jacqui stares into her drink, looking hopeless for a moment. I know she won't accept money from me for private healthcare, as I've asked her again tonight and she said no again.

'Nothing, nothing. Just be there for me, like you always are. Listen, I'm tired. I'm going to call it a night, if that's okay.'

'Of course,' I say.

We book taxis and hug each other in the street before going our separate ways. I worry about Jacqui, with the world's woes on her shoulders. My problems are nothing compared to hers. A sick child is the fucking pits, I can see that.

When I get home and I've sobered up a bit, I read the email we sent to Clio to find that it is coherent and not ill-advised, though of course it was a dumb idea to send it when we were pissed. We got away with it though. Then I write myself a note to message Tara tomorrow and get a meeting sorted with her too. After my talk with Jacqui tonight, I'm not really any the wiser about what's going on with Clio. Maybe it's nothing. Maybe Jacqui's suspicions are baseless. Maybe everything is fine. At least I can sleep tonight with this thought (and the help of several pornstar martinis).

Chapter 22

On Monday morning, I get a reply from Clio. She agrees to the meeting and we set a date in a couple of weeks. That's not ideal for me – I want to get this sorted sooner! But she's evasive and says she's fully booked up till then. I've offered for the meeting to take place at my office, but then Clio says she'd rather it be at her house and presents that as a done deal. I think it might be a power move, and that makes me feel weird about her again. But I'm not going to fight about it and create a bad feeling.

I spent most of yesterday in bed, as I was so worn out after my drinking session with Jac. I did a lot of googling and I watched a couple of TV documentaries. I found out about cancer scammers. Oh. My. Fucking. God. The nerve of these people! The lies upon lies upon lies. They told not only their social media followers that they had cancer when they didn't, but also their friends, their families. Their own children! They paid visits to A&E (or the emergency room or whatever they call it elsewhere) and took photos of themselves pretending to be ill, while the hospitals had to agree to see them, as they didn't know if they were lying or not. Then posted it as cancer treatment. Others bought medical equipment online and staged faked photos of themselves at home surrounded by the paraphernalia of illness to pretend they were having chemo or other treatments. Some did it just for attention, others for money – not just cash donations to GoFundMe accounts to spend on extra holidays and jewellery or whatever, but they based their businesses on their cancer experiences, so got book deals and app deals and all sorts of kickbacks and advantages, all the while praised and supported by an army of online followers, most of whom had never met them and yet were deeply into warm, parasocial relationships with these 'brave' women who'd fought cancer and won. The lengths people will go to in order to steal money instead of working their arses off like the rest of us – it will never cease to amaze me. Google them yourself, if you want to know more. It'll blow your mind. These utter fuckers have no shame, honestly. So, now I'm wondering, is Clio one of these? Could she possibly be? She hasn't used social media at all. She doesn't have an international reach. It's all very local and low-key. But just look at how nice her pretty barn conversion is. Look at the prices she's charging for her retreats, her sessions, her products she must get affiliate earnings for (considering how hard she pushed them) and also, her charities. At least they're getting something out of it, I suppose. But at what cost? The truth? And therein lies the problem: I still don't know what the truth is. And that's why I need to talk to Tara.

Tara also gets back to me on Monday. We agree to go to a wine bar near the office straight from work. We walk together, gossip a bit about work and then I ask after her sons and we talk about their comings and goings until we're sitting in a booth with a glass of red wine each.

'Something tells me this meeting over wine isn't just about work, or my kids. There's something on your mind,' says Tara, astutely. She's no fool.

'Yes, you're right. I need to ask you about something. It's about Clio.'

Tara looks intrigued. 'Okay . . . '

'About Clio's cancer. I wondered if she'd discussed it with you at all.'

'Well, yes, she did.'

There's a pregnant pause.

'I wondered what Clio said to you about her cancer.'

Tara pauses again. She seems to be considering something.

'The truth is that we . . . well, we did discuss it at length.'

That's a promising start.

Tara goes on, 'Because . . . well, firstly, this must remain confidential.'

What's this?

'Of course,' I say, my HR hat suddenly landing on my head. 'And you don't have to say anything. We can stop this conversation right now.'

'No, it's okay. I think it's probably about time I mention this. The reason I discussed Clio's cancer with her is because I've been through it myself.'

Oh God, I did not foresee this for one second.

'Oh Tara, I had no idea.'

'Of course you didn't. Because I don't tell people about it. Especially not at work. I don't want people thinking I'm flaky.'

'How could anyone think that?!'

Tara raises her eyebrows. 'You'd be surprised. Especially some men I've come across at work. They think breast cancer means there's something innately wrong with you as a woman.'

'Surely not. That would be outrageous.'

'It's not a rational thing. And it's never said. But at my last place of work, when I was going through it, I definitely got that impression. They couldn't sack me. But I knew the male management treated me differently afterwards. Like I was damaged goods.'

'Jesus, that's horrible. I don't think even the tactless Derek would act that way.'

'Let's hope not. But that's why I haven't disclosed it at work. There's no need to, of course. I've been fine for a while now. But yes, that's why Clio helped me so much with it. I had breast cancer five years ago. I had a lumpectomy and radiotherapy and went into remission. And it helped me so much to know that Clio had also beaten breast cancer.'

Breast? Clio had *breast* cancer? So Clio had cervical, bowel, thyroid and now breast cancer *as well*? Oh Christ, she *is* a scammer. Surely she is. Surely this is a step too far. How the hell am I going to handle this? How am I going to support Tara with what she just told me, as well as simultaneously finding out what I need to know? But the fact remains that I don't know that much about these other cancers. I researched the hell out of lung cancer for my dad, of course. I'm an expert in that club that I never wanted to belong to. But these other cancers . . . I just don't know enough about how they metastasise. And I will have to tread very, very carefully with Tara about this, now I know she's been through it herself.

'I'm so sorry to hear this, Tara. Truly sorry, that you had

to go through that. And so glad to hear you're doing so well now.'

'Thanks, I appreciate that.'

'And it will of course remain completely confidential.'

'Good. Thanks again.'

There's an awkward silence. Even though we've bonded this past week, the truth is that I don't know this woman at all really and she doesn't know me either. There's a question hanging in the air about where this conversation is going next and I don't know who is going to ask that question. Or who's going to answer it. My gut feeling is telling me to leave this topic alone, now I've found out that Tara has gone through this horrible disease. At the very least, I should be leaving a period of time in between finding out about Tara's disease and pursuing this subject as relates to Clio. So that's what I decide to do. I'm going to change the subject.

'But why were you asking about Clio's cancer?' Tara says suddenly.

And there it is. The point of no return. If I try to make out some bullshit fudging answer, Tara will see straight through it. I've got to try though.

'No reason, really. I was just interested in it.'

'Sure,' says Tara, though her face doesn't look at all sure. She looks suspicious. 'But you asked me just now, specifically, what Clio had told me *about* her cancer. Why did you ask that?'

There's no getting one over Tara.

'Okay . . . so, the facts are that she's told different people that she had different cancers.'

May as well just come out with it now. Cards on the table. Tara is too smart to hoodwink.

'Which ones?'

Tara's face is a mask. Mental note to never play her at poker.

'She told me she had cervical cancer. Then she's told other clients she had bowel cancer and thyroid cancer. And now she told you breast cancer.'

Tara's mask slips, for a fraction of a second. There's a definite twitch there. But she betrays no other emotion.

'Who, exactly, did she tell this to?'

Tara is coming at it now as a legal expert. So I try to be as factual as possible.

'She told the daughter of the folk who run Roseland Hall that she had bowel cancer. She told me cervical. She told a woman at the retreat that I spoke to that she had thyroid cancer. Each of these people had close relatives who had had these cancers and Clio, it turned out, had had all of the same cancers too. She also told me that she'd received treatment in one hospital, whereas she told the others that she had been treated in a different hospital. She also told me she had a sister and left home at sixteen and never looked back, whereas she told the woman I spoke to that she had one brother and cut ties with her family five years ago.'

There are the bald facts. I'm waiting for Tara to respond. But again, that poker face is impressive. Then, finally, Tara speaks.

'Clio had cancer in both breasts. UCLH told her they'd have to do a double mastectomy but she refused and did her own treatment instead and kept her breasts. She went into remission and made a full recovery.'

'UCLH?'

'Yes, in London.'

'Tara, she told me she was at Maidstone Hospital. Charles Dickens centre, I remember the conversation distinctly.'

'Cancer can often be a complex disease,' says Tara testily. 'People can end up being treated at different hospitals for different aspects of the condition.'

'I can see that. But . . . that's four different types now – cervical, bowel, thyroid and breast. Maybe it spread. Can it spread from breast to cervical to bowel and even to thyroid? I'm not sure. I don't think it's very common to spread to the thyroid from those other areas of the body and – even if it did – surely nutrition alone couldn't cure that? She'd be extremely seriously sick.'

'Well, that just shows how well she did to recover fully,' says Tara, with a note of finality.

There's another silence and I'm rapidly considering which way to proceed as I stare into the depths of my wine.

Tara intervenes. 'What exactly are you trying to suggest, Lucy?'

I look up at her. She doesn't look worried. She looks suspicious. She looks defensive. Oh God, the fact may well be that – if Clio is a liar – she's done quite a number on Tara, another sufferer whose deeply distressing experience Clio has used to her own advantage, if that is indeed the case. Unless this whole thing is a massive misunderstanding borne from Jacqui's spidey senses and the two of us drinking too many cocktails.

'The truth is I don't know what I'm suggesting, not really. But . . . doesn't it strike you as weird that Clio has told everyone a different story about her cancer? And other details of her life.'

'No, I think she told people the bit that affected them, that was relevant to them. Maybe she didn't want it to become a competition, as in, you've had breast cancer? Is that all? Well, I've had breast and thyroid and pancreatic and all sorts, so I win!' Tara laughs scoffingly.

'Not pancreatic,' I reply, wanting to keep things factual. 'Bowel. And cervical. My grandmother had cervical. It doesn't strike you as quite the coincidence that Clio just happened to have suffered from the exact same cancers as each of her clients or their relatives?'

'No,' says Tara emphatically. 'No, it does not. Clio is an incredibly intuitive person. It's very likely these clients were drawn to her and she to them because of this link between them.'

Now, that's the first time in this conversation that Tara has gone off the boil with her razor-sharp analysis.

'How could anyone intuit that someone has had cancer in a particular part of their body?'

'There are many things that we can't explain by pure science,' says Tara and starts fiddling with the stem of her wine glass. The wine is sloshing a bit in the glass, threatening to spill over on to the white cloth we have at this table in the window of the wine bar. Then, Tara's tone completely changes. 'Look, this is very unfair to Clio. Don't you think the poor woman has been through enough? She got me through the aftermath of my cancer because she knew *exactly* what it was like to go through it herself. If I hadn't met Clio I don't think I'd still be with my husband, because she made me realise the reason I wanted to escape was because I had undiagnosed PTSD from my breast cancer. We worked through it all together. She knew all the feelings about that fear of losing your breasts, the effect on your femininity. She understood it all. You can't fake that.'

259

Now we get to the crux of the matter. I can see the deep effect Clio has had on Tara. And how much she's helped her. Who am I to interfere with that, whatever the truth is? This whole conversation has been a mistake. I see that now.

'I'm so sorry, Tara, about this whole thing. I should never have asked you about it. I can only apologise. Let's end this here. I think it's for the best.'

'No, because I'm not done yet.'

That's fighting talk. A couple nearby glance at us and I'm starting to feel really uncomfortable. Maybe I should just get up and take my leave. But Tara is going full steam ahead.

'What exactly are you saying about Clio and her cancer then? Say precisely what you're implying.'

My heart is beating harder now. It's at times like this you can see what a good litigator Tara is, especially now I'm bearing the brunt of this. I could cave. I could pretend she's won and I was wrong. But now I've heard that Clio told her all that stuff about having breast cancer as well, the truth is I'm more convinced than ever that there is something very wrong going on. And hearing Tara's experiences makes me even more determined to find out the truth, because my heart goes out to her, however much she's gunning for me right now. I recognise her defensiveness. It's like a rerun of me and Jacqui, except this time, I'm the one seeing sense.

'I'm starting to consider the possibility that Clio might never have had cancer at all and has lied about the whole thing for personal gain.'

'What? That's ridiculous!'

Tara laughs like a shout. But there's something in her eyes that wants explanation.

'Is it though, Tara? It's happened before throughout time,

grifters lying about their health and touting miracle cures. Snake oil salesmen and the like. And more recently, it's still happening. Modern-day scammers using social media to lie to their followers for more sympathy and thus more likes and follows and influence and money, yes, money.'

Tara goes very quiet. Then she looks me dead in the eye.

'I won't hear baseless accusations against her. This is slander.'

'I know. That's why I wanted to talk to someone else who'd worked with Clio and see what she said to them. I had no idea you'd had cancer yourself, Tara. If I'd known, I'd never have asked you about it.'

'You think it makes me weak? Makes me lack judgement?'

'God, no! No! Absolutely not. But if Clio has been lying to everyone about having cancer, don't you think we need to do something about it? Morally, if for no other reason?'

'Ah, but there is another reason, isn't there?'

What's this? The argument has become really heated now. People are looking. And since this could well be slander, we probably shouldn't be discussing this at all in public. Christ, this is a bloody mess. But what is she talking about now?

'I don't know what you mean, Tara, and frankly, I think this discussion should be over. It's not getting us anywhere.'

Tara has that look on her face, the exact same way she looked at me when she accused me of lying about the wellness stuff to impress our bosses. She was right then, however nastily she said it. But what is she suggesting now?

'Not yet. The truth is, if Clio is a scammer, you're in a hell of a lot of trouble at work. You're the one who's lauded her most to the CEOs. It's not me who's hired Clio to be the keynote speaker. If it comes out that she's fraudulent, the CEOs won't think too highly of you. However, I can sidestep it easily, retreat from having any knowledge of it, and make sure I am the one who is in no way to blame. This conference is your baby. So, if I were you, I'd stop attacking a dear woman who has saved many lives and many people's sanity, including mine. And think about your own problems. Because if this blows up, it'll take you with it.'

With that, Tara shoves her wine glass away and the red liquid sloshes over the edge, finally free, blooming across the white tablecloth like a wound. She grabs her handbag and marches out of there, leaving me sitting alone with my red wine, which I proceed to drink down in one like Ribena on school sports day.

That went well.

Chapter 23

Everything is worse after that meeting. Now that Tara and I have had a big fallout, it won't be easy at work. And now she thinks I'm being slanderous about someone who saved her. Part of me wishes I'd never had these doubts. Part of me just wants Clio to be this shining presence in our lives again, instead of a fraud. But once you suspect something like that, it niggles at you. It's the pea under the mattresses. And it doesn't take a princess to work out that there's something potentially very dodgy about Clio Kenton.

Tara really has drunk the Kool-Aid and there's no talking her round, not yet anyway, and not without any concrete evidence. And, deep down, I don't want Clio to be a scammer. I want to be back in the warm embrace of the pool of light that formed around Clio, that fell on anyone in her near radius. And now I'm out in the cold, it feels awful. I'm beginning to hate Clio for that, for shutting me out, so suddenly. Maybe she lied about the cancer, her childhood, but she still helped me. All the requests for money and the app and links to buy stuff – I mean she has to make a living but she doesn't need to leech off her clients that badly, does she? But I just have this horrible, growing conviction that I've been scammed by Clio, just like all the credulous idiots I used to laugh at who believed in various other wellness grifters. I mean, what if the cancer money isn't even going to the cancer charities? I can see now I've been on a kind of addictive high and I'm only now coming back down to earth. The only way I'm going to work any of this out is if I do my research on her. Project Clio: true or false?

My biggest problem now is the staff conference in just over three weeks' time. What the hell am I going to do? If I cancel Clio, Derek will think I've made a bad error of judgement. Clio might even make it difficult for me, make it legally a problem, demanding payment anyway. Derek would never agree to that and it'd make me look really bad in front of the new CEO Nick Bridges, especially since Tara will say that Clio is legit and I'm being ridiculous trying to cancel her.

What I need is proof. What I need is to investigate and find the proof I require. What I need is an investigator. What I need is . . . Jacqui.

That Monday night, home exhausted after the showdown with Tara and finally ensconced on the sofa, I message Jacqui.

Well, that was a fucking disaster. Turns out Tara had breast cancer and Clio told her she had breast cancer too. And Tara won't hear a bad word against her. I don't know what to do next, honey. I really don't. Any ideas, oh wise one??

Jacqui doesn't answer straight away, so I pour myself another glass of red and order a Domino's. Only a small pepperoni plus sides of spicy chicken wings and coleslaw are going to assuage my worries tonight.

Then I get a reply from Jacqui.

You bet your bottom dollar I'm the wise one. And yeah, I have an idea. In fact, I've already started. You seem to have forgotten you have a best pal who is also an investigative journalist. Well, I've been on the case since Sunday morning. I was just waiting till tonight to confirm something and now I have, so it's time to dish the dirt. Have I got some little bits of shit on our Clio to shovel for you!

This is followed by a grinning devil emoji.

Oh my fucking god! What??!!

Easier to explain face to face. Got time for a video chat right now?

I immediately tap on the camera icon and Jacqui answers. And she's grinning.

'What? What?? Whaaat?!' I cry. 'What have you found out?'

'Tell me about this meeting with Tara first.'

I explain what happened briefly and how rotten all round it was.

'Well, she'll have to come round when she hears this lot. And I'm convinced this is only the beginning. Okay. Ready?'

'Fuck YES. Get on with it, woman.'

'Right, first of all, I want you to tell me everything you know about Clio. Start at the beginning, tell me everything she told you.'

'But I want to hear the shit you've shovelled first!'

'Nope, I need your testimony first. To check against some of the things I've found out, make sure they fit.'

So, I tell Jacqui everything I can think of – about her leaving her mother and sister and home at sixteen and never looking back, being diagnosed with cervical cancer in 2021, trying treatment then stopping it, then healing herself through nutrition. Then starting as a wellness practitioner, plus the two charities she helps on her website. That's everything I can think of.

'Now dish it!'

'Okay, so I've only been looking into it for a couple of days, but I've found out a couple of things so far. So, her name isn't Clio Kenton. It's a business name. Her real name is Julia Dorian-Vincent.'

'Wow, that's a mouthful. Sounds posh too.'

'You're not wrong. Turns out Julia D-V has had several business names over the last ten years or so. Clio Kenton is only the latest. Once I found out her real name, I was able to find two other businesses so far. One was selling essential oils and handmade candles as Sabrina Fox, back in 2015 for two years, in St Leonards-on-Sea, East Sussex. Another was offering something called 'spiritual massage' in 2018 as Luna Michelle, over in Southend-on-Sea in Essex. That business ended in 2020. Since then, she's set up as Clio Kenton in early 2020 – just before the pandemic hit – and has been doing this past-life regression business from her home here as Clarity with Clio.'

'All of that sounds a bit scammy. And she sure gets about

a bit. And she likes the on-Sea suffixes. But it's not illegal, as far as we know.'

'No, anyone can change their name, of course. Okay, so there's more. I rang the two cancer charities on her website who she claims to represent and collect donations for. Now, here's the really juicy bit: one of the charities, the Polly Twelvetrees one, says that Clio did some publicity with them once for their website and gave them a bit of money. But nothing since then.'

'How long ago was that?'

'Erm . . . that was in 2022. And the other one – the Cancer Kids one – said she did a fundraiser event with them in . . . 2023 . . . but she's paid them nothing since.'

'Fucking hell. And she's still taking money in their name. The charity direct debit goes to Clio's account.'

'Is that definite, that she's still taking money she claims is for them?' asks Jacqui, pencil paused above her notes.

'Yes, definitely. She mentioned them both by name at the weekend retreat.'

'Okay, good. They're on her website, but she could always claim it's out of date. But if she's still mentioning them by name in her class, then that's more evidence.'

This is sounding bad, very bad. I try to think of alternative explanations, other than the obvious one of charity fraud. 'Is it possible the person you spoke to just didn't know? Or wasn't allowed to go through a list of donors?'

'It is possible, yeah. I left my name with both of them, telling them about Clio's website and the payments she's taken on their behalf. So we'll see if they get in touch. And that's everything I've found out, for now. But believe me, chick, I've only just begun.'

I feel a bit sick. So, Clio is really Julia – or Sabrina or Luna. She's not Clio, anyway. All of that is fake. And her story about starting wellness after she got cancer in 2021 is not true either, as she was at it back in 2015 onwards. And this news from the charities, that they've not even heard from her in two years.

'This isn't looking good,' I say glumly.

'I know . . . ' says Jacqui and looks at me, clearly worried about me.

'But nothing's proven yet,' I say, trying to remain bright. 'After all, a person can change their name and business. It doesn't mean they're a liar. And the cancer charities might just have been misinformed, i.e. you could've been talking to a minion who didn't know anything. Or couldn't share information about donations.'

'True, true. Look, I want to carry on investigating. Are you okay with that?'

'Are you thinking about writing an article about this then?'

'I am, yeah. I don't think the boss will be able to turn this one down. Not since local residents will have been taken in by Clio Kenton. But I must have all my ducks in a row first, before I approach him. And there's definitely more to uncover, I bet. But, I would only pursue it if I have the go-ahead from you. The last thing I want to do is make trouble for you. I could leave it until well after the conference has come and gone. I mean, it's only three weeks away, yeah? Or I could leave it altogether, Lu. Just forget I ever heard a thing about it. If that makes life easier for you. You're my priority, not this woman and her dodgy ways.'

I consider this for a moment. If Jacqui drops it, then it could all go away. We do the conference, with Clio as our guest speaker – who I'm sure will go down a storm, as everyone loves her as a speaker – and then I impress Derek and Nick, and I get the promotion (fingers crossed) and I never see Clio again. It could all work out like that.

'I . . . just don't know. I don't know what to do.'

Jacqui can see I'm conflicted. She smiles kindly at me and says, 'Listen, don't worry. I can leave it all here. Is that what you'd rather I do? Or I can keep on investigating and tell you what I find out. And after that, it's up to you what you do with that information. And I will abide by whatever decision you make. As I said, you – and our friendship – are my priorities.'

I look at Jacqui and – not for the first time – I feel so lucky she's my best mate.

'Thank you so much, darling,' I say. 'The truth is, I've no idea what to do for the best. But also, I want to know what the truth is. I have to. It's eating me up inside. And whatever I decide to do about the conference, the fact is that I need to know for my own personal satisfaction, what the truth is about Clio. Or whatever the fuck her name is.'

'Okay, deal. I'll keep sniffing around. And I'll feed back to you whatever I find out. We've got three weeks till the conference. Let's see what I can unearth, eh?'

I thank Jacqui and we finish our video call. Then I sit in a slump on the sofa for an age. Well, until the Domino's lady rings my doorbell and then I again sit on my sofa in a slump, but this time I have pizza and spicy wings for company, at least. I'm in shock, to tell the truth. Hearing that Clio had all these businesses in different names – and Clio isn't even her name – has left a bad taste in my mouth, not even ameliorated by creamy coleslaw or a swig of wine. Jacqui has been brilliant, as ever. And she's also been lovely and very understanding. This could be a great story for her. And she's promised me she won't share it unless or until I agree. That is beyond kindness. She wants the best for me. But my fear is that the cat is already out of the bag. By speaking to those charities, I'm guessing that whoever took those calls may well start asking questions. And once that happens, if Clio is up to no good, then the truth will out, eventually. But maybe there was a misunderstanding. Or even if there weren't, then maybe whoever took those calls won't bother about it.

But can I live with finding out Clio is a scammer and keep it all quiet, to protect my chances of getting my long-sought promotion? To let her carry on, lying to clients, pretending to have cancer to screw more money out of them, exploiting their own cancer experiences and their vulnerability to line her pockets? As a moral dilemma, it's a doozy. But, despite all the evidence piling up, we still have no definitive proof that she's lied about anything. It could all be circumstantial. Clio could be perfectly legit. There is still hope.

Chapter 24

The following week and a half goes by in a lumpy, bumpy way, as Tara isn't talking to me at work and I'm trying to draw together resources and ideas for my conference speech and PowerPoint, while also trying to impress Derek and Nick Bridges, the latter attending more regularly now his handover with Derek is imminent. The day of the conference will be Derek's last and Nick's official first and it's when they'll announce the new COO. Both Tara and I have had informal discussions with both Derek and Nick about the COO post and all of that's been logged. The gossip on the street (or around the office water cooler) is that it's too close to call: Tara's wow factor as new blood is equally matched by my deep knowledge of the business. So, it's anyone's guess who'll win the promotion.

In the meantime, I'm constantly waiting to hear back from Jacqui, who hasn't had anything to report about her Clio investigations since that heady Sunday night more than a week ago. She says she'll only tell me stuff when she's had things confirmed from more than one source, so as not to muddy the waters. Fair enough. But my God, I'm gagging to know more. And all of a sudden, the evening of the meeting with Clio is here and I'm still no closer to knowing the truth. I've come home from work, showered, washed my hair, blow-dried it straight and neat, and changed into a fresh suit, my best grey suit that actually makes me look pretty natty. (I know that using the word 'natty' automatically signals me as not natty at all, i.e. hopelessly out of touch. But I feel good anyway.) I want to look my most professional for this crucial meeting, largely because – and I'm not exaggerating – I'm shitting myself about it. (Just spent the last half-hour on the loo. Thank God for Imodium Instants – but do they really work that fast? Or do they make you think they're working and then that calms you down and you don't feel so anxious and that stops you having the shits? Placebo effect there again, you see. It's not only the wellness industry that uses it: so does the illness industry . . .)

I'm just about to leave when my phone starts ringing.

'Who the *fuck* is that?' I say aloud, which is what I always say on the rare occasion my phone rings or even my doorbell. My stomach lurches as I presume it must be Clio cancelling the meeting last minute on some thin pretext. But actually, it's Jacqui.

'Hey,' I say.

'Hey you.'

'I'm literally this second leaving for Clio's.'

'I'm glad I caught you then. Just found something that might be useful.'

'Hit me!'

'Okay, so Clio's background. Or rather, Julia Dorian-

Vincent's. She has two brothers. I'm trying to track them down currently and don't have any more confirmed info on them. But what I have established without doubt is that she is very much in touch with her parents. The barn conversion with the bare stone walls is in their name and she's living there as she has lasting power of attorney for both her parents. They currently live in a very expensive care home near Dover. I had a chat with the caretaker, who hates working there and he dished some dirt for me. He says she visits once a year, on New Year's Day and that's it. They've been there for ten years apparently, one suffering from Alzheimer's and the other bed-bound, so they're in a pretty bad way.'

I feel a lump in my throat and then swallow it down. It was a big lump of guilt. I haven't visited Mum in New Zealand at all. Not once. Yes, we've done video calls but I haven't seen her face to face since she and Shirl left, six years ago. Am I a bad daughter? Am I as neglectful as Clio Kenton – or Julia Whats-her-name? Well, in my defence, Dover is a tad nearer than the antipodes.

Jacqui continues, 'The caretaker was most forthcoming! I think actually he fancied me a bit. We shared a cigarette. He said he's been there since leaving school and he's in his thirties now and all he wanted to be in life was a chartered surveyor – I mean, weird ambition, but hey – so I told him he should be a chartered surveyor if he really wants to and fuck this crappy job. There, I'm his life coach now.'

I laugh and say, 'That's great information, thanks, love.' But 'chartered surveyor' . . . that's reminding me of something . . .

'Well, Clio has certainly lied about having a sister. There's no record of any sister that I can find.'

'Okay. Right, thanks so much for that. I must get off. I'll let you know what I find out. Oh and by the way, it just occurs to me that there's something I forgot to mention and that's that Clio said that before she got into the wellness industry, she said she was a chartered surveyor. I forgot to tell you that and your caretaker's lofty ambition just reminded me. Yeah, she definitely said she used to be a chartered surveyor. Might be another lie but an odd thing to lie about. Not exactly a flex.'

'Ooh, that's good. Okay, I'll get on to that. Good luck with the meeting from hell! I mean, sorry. What I meant to say was, give her hell!'

Honestly, I feel sick as a dog. I have to deal with confrontation all the time at work, daily at times. And it rarely, if ever, fazes me. But confrontation outside of work – especially with someone as clever as Clio – makes me go all wobbly and breathless. Plus, I'd be lying to myself if I don't admit that I'm excited to see her again. I've missed her presence in my life. I hate that she has that over me. But what I'm hoping against hope is that tonight, Clio can explain everything and put all my fears to rest. And then everything will be fine.

God, I hope so.

When I get to her house, she's dressed casually yet coolly in pale green denims and a cute grey hoodie with a dolphin and Marine Conservation Society on it and I wonder if she's scamming them too. I feel overdressed. Oh well, hopefully my attire will signal to Clio that I mean business. And I most certainly do. Clio shows me through the exposed stone wall of her hallway (I mean it looks lovely, but I've always wondered about those kinds of walls, if they just gather dust and spiders in large quantities). We go through to her therapy

274

room, even though we're not doing therapy today (I hope not anyway. I want to be in charge, not her). She's all smiles and professionalism, asking how work is going, how my mother is, my sister and her family. I keep my replies short and resist the urge to ask how she is, as I would usually politely do with anyone. I have to keep my feelings out of this. Tonight I'm all business.

Clio sits in her usual therapist's chair and has put out a similar chair for me, so at least I'm not stuck on the couch feeling like a patient. I start formally with a question about her speech that she'll be giving at the staff conference exactly two weeks today – what it's going to be about, what it'll contain, what the message is.

'My focus will be the wellness of your staff and what measures they can take personally and professionally to self-optimise. They'll be user-friendly suggestions – no hint of bootcamps or anything like that. It'll be simple things mostly, like making time for themselves, grounding themselves, walking in fresh air, seeing people and places that give them joy. And there will also be some advice on treating themselves kindly, as they would treat someone they cared for, rather than someone they might neglect or even dislike. My message will be that in order to shine as a person at home and in the world, your priority has to be yourself and your own wellness, for if we're suffering under a depletion of our own wellness, how can we possibly help others achieve their own greatness? That's about the size of it. How does that sound?'

It sounds great. I mean, there's a risk of it verging a little on the woo-woo side, but knowing how smart Clio is, I'm sure it won't and it'll be down-to-earth and brilliant, as she ever was. And then I just feel rotten, because all of my faith in her and my admiration for her has been tainted forever by what I know.

'That sounds very good, thank you. So, I have a few questions from management that we just need clearing up before we go ahead,' I lie. Well, it's a white lie. I am management and I am asking the questions so . . . yeah.

'Sure,' she says in an accommodating tone, wrapping one leg around the other in an effortless, yoga-style way. I feel stiff as a board and awkward as hell.

'So, as regards your health. You've talked openly about your experiences with cancer.'

I pause. This all feels wrong. But I must persevere. This might be my only chance.

I continue. 'Did you have more than one type of cancer?'

She looks shocked. But immediately, her face rearranges itself. She's good at that.

'Yes, I did. It metastasised.'

'So, which cancers did you have?'

I'm pretending to write notes down but it's all for show. I'm finding it difficult to meet her gaze – that intense blue gaze she uses on you, to get you to stop thinking.

'I suffered with cervical cancer which metastasised to several others.'

'Which ones, precisely?'

'A range,' is all she'd say.

'Skin cancer was one of them, yes?'

I throw that in as a spanner. But she doesn't rise to it.

'No, not skin cancer.'

'So, you visited multiple hospitals.'

'Yes, you know what a lottery the NHS is. I was treated by different specialists at different hospitals.'

276

'Which hospitals were you treated at?'

'There were so many. I can't recall them all.'

I snap my eyes up from my pen.

'You can't remember which hospitals you were treated at?'

'All right, there was Maidstone Hospital. And UCLH.'

'Any others?'

I know the Royal Marsden was one she told Bitsy.

'I can't recall. It was four years ago. And I have tried to block out a lot of it. It's due to the PTSD I suffered as a result of my cancer and the medieval treatments imposed upon me. Sometimes I have blanks in my memory.'

Good answer, I'm thinking. Perfect excuse. I need to counter it.

'And the Chaucer Hospital.'

I throw that in there. It's in Canterbury but nobody said she went there. It's a little test for our Clio.

'No, not that one. I've never heard of that one.'

Dammit. I was hoping she'd fall for that trap.

'Royal Marsden?' I say and she nods immediately.

'Yes, I went to that one.'

This isn't getting me anywhere. I move on.

'So, you eschewed formal medical treatment and took your own path. Can you explain, how exactly did you cure yourself? How did that work when you had multiple cancers all over your body?'

Clio sighs, as if listening to a child. I'm starting to feel more and more tetchy now. And *eschewed* is a damn good word. But Clio is outpacing me at every step.

'We all have the power to heal ourselves. If you'd stayed with my therapy, then we'd have got on to that down our path. But unfortunately, you decided to mix business with therapy and now we can't. I'm sorry but that was your decision. I have to be very careful who I work with. I've been burnt in the past.'

That was a jibe directly aimed. At me. Plus she hasn't explained anything of how she actually cured her cancer.

'But what techniques did you use? Specifically?'

'Three techniques: nutrition, nutrition and nutrition.'

Urgh, don't echo Tony Blair. His PR isn't so great these days.

'And how does that work, exactly?'

'As I've said, I would've got on to that with you in our therapy. But I don't share that information for free. The recipes on the app will give you some idea but that's not the full story. Through my therapy, I would share the rest with you. But, as I say, that's something that only my clients have access to.'

Hmm, she's getting snippy now. Maybe I'm getting under her skin a little, tiny bit. Let's push it a little further.

'You work with two cancer charities, is that right?'

'I help them out, yes.'

'Have you sent all of that charity money given by your clients and website visitors to those cancer charities?'

I thought that would make her gulp. But she goes straight into her answer seamlessly. God, she's good. Ovaries of steel.

'I manage my cash flow how I see fit. It all goes into the same pot. I have to control the money coming in and out according to need. The charities will and do receive their payments, of course, when the time is right. That's my business model and it works for me.'

That's a smart answer. And impossible to mess with really. I'm running out of ammo. I'm going to have to go personal.

'Okay and lastly, your family. You've mentioned a sister, that you left home at sixteen and never looked back. Yet you've also mentioned a brother and how you decided to walk away from your family at the beginning of the pandemic. So, there are some confusing stories out there and it would be useful if you could clarify the truth, so we can accurately construct a bio for you.'

Now she looks pissed off.

'I shouldn't have to remind you that my professional life is separate from my personal life and despite the fact that I am providing a paid service for you and your company, I still have a right to privacy. I feel, Lucy, that you've managed to collate some random bits of information about me and all you're doing is trying to construct a whole picture from fragments. And to be honest with you, I'm really not convinced that your colleagues at work want to know all of this stuff about me. I feel rather that these questions are coming from you personally. And really it's all quite upsetting, being quizzed like this by someone I felt I had such a good rapport with. Didn't you feel that too, Lu?'

I'm thinking, *Yes, yes, I did. I thought you were the best fucking thing since sliced bread.* But I'm not telling her that now, not now. I mustn't let my feelings get the better of me.

'Yes, I did. But I am concerned about the conflicting versions of your illness and your life that you have made public and all I am doing is seeking to nail down the facts. I'm doing my due diligence as a director of Beane & Co.'

Clio looks down at that moment. She raises her hands and presses her index fingers to her temples, as if trying to avert a migraine. It's all very effective acting. For now, I can honestly say, I'm sure that's what it is. Then, she looks up suddenly. Her voice sounds different, strained.

'I feel you're being very unfair. And the truth is that I really cannot deal with all this right now. As I mentioned in my recent email, there has been a crisis I'm dealing with in recent weeks. And all of this – all these intrusive questions – is not helping one bit. Because . . . well . . . I suppose I'm going to have to tell you this, because otherwise you won't stop haranguing me. But the truth is, if you must know, the cancer has come back.'

Pause. Dramatic tension. She's staring me down with those piercing blue eyes, willing me to say how shocked and sorry I am. But I don't say that.

I say, 'The cancer has come back?'

She replies, with a halting voice, 'Yes, I'm afraid so. My cancer has come back.'

'Which *one*?' I say.

She looks at me with faked sadness. I'm sure it's fake. I'm sure the cancer coming back is fake. I'm sure the whole damn persona is fake.

'All of them, if you must know. And this time, nutrition won't be the answer, I'm afraid. I'll need surgery. And hospitalisation.'

She sounds like she's about to cry. But I feel nothing. Absolutely nothing.

'What kind of surgery?'

'That really is none of your business!' she says and wipes a fake tear from her eye.

She thinks I'll fold if she raises her voice at me. But I'm used to troublesome people shouting at me. And I'm in work mode now. Her feigned righteous anger doesn't bother me in the slightest.

'All right then. Something that is my business is if you are able to fulfil the contract you've signed with us for the conference speech. When is the surgery?' I ask.

She recovers herself remarkably and says, 'A week after our conference. I'll be going in for various tests before that, but I'll be okay. Don't worry, I'll be at the conference. I will fulfil our contract. And now, I'm sorry, I am very tired and I need to rest. The cancers are eating up my energy, I'm afraid. It really is time for you to go.'

There's nothing more to do here. I'm done. I've asked everything I wanted to ask. And she's hedged and obfuscated and finally, played the sympathy card. And despite having no firm proof either way, I'm now one hundred per cent certain that Clio Kenton – or Julia D-V – is an out and out liar.

'Of course. And don't get up, Clio. You need your rest. See you on Friday 28th at the cinema. We've booked out a theatre there for the conference and there will be food. I'm not sure it'll live up to your wellness standards, I'm afraid. Our workforce prefers mini beef burgers and Death by Chocolate to green juices, I'm sorry to say. Here's hoping your speech converts them. I'll see myself out.'

I walk past her to the door and leave. I don't look back. I don't want to. The thought of seeing Clio Kenton again and her lying face makes me feel sick. You think I'm being too hard on her? You think there's a chance she's legit? That she really did have all those cancers and cured herself? And now, the tragic woman has to deal with the cancer returning, after all the heroic efforts she's made to beat it? Well, you weren't in the room with me. And I'm telling you, the look on her face when she told me the cancer had come back – it was triumph. Pure, unadulterated victory. Because she knew she was spotless, unable to be touched, scot-free from all responsibility, because she had cancer again and there was nothing I could say to disprove it. I can still see Dad's face when he was told his cancer had metastasised. When he knew that the worst was not over, for the worst was yet to come. And it wasn't triumph. It wasn't victory. It was fear. And despair.

Fuck Clio Kenton and her despicable lies. She's on my fucking shit list now.

Chapter 25

The week of the conference arrives and my time leading up to this week has been filled with hours of research and writing my conference speech and nothing new at all from Jacqui on Clio the scammer. I need more hard evidence of Clio being a liar before I can decide what to do next. Bad vibes won't cut it when it comes to trying to cancel a contract and deal with the inevitable backlash from the CEOs. I'm going to need something more damning and Jacqui is still looking and researching, bless her. And I'm tearing my hair out waiting. So, today I'm at work and all the directors plus the outgoing CEO Derek and the CEO-to-be Nick are discussing the staff conference coming up at the end of this week. Right now, through gritted teeth, I'm having to listen to both Derek and Nick banging on about Clio's speech and how much they're looking forward to it, while Tara is waxing lyrical about Clio and saying how she's still seeing her regularly for therapy and it's mind-blowing and how it's totally changed her outlook on life and even Derek is going on about how impressed he is with Clio's ideas. Then Nick says how he's so impressed that the whole staff conference will be focused on workplace wellness and how innovative that is, with Clio as their star speaker.

Nick adds, 'Looking forward to your speech too, obviously, Lucia.' (Oh God, Nick is calling me Lucia now as well. For fuck's sake!) 'And Tara's speech, of course.'

Tara's what?!

I ask, in a neutral voice, 'Tara's giving a speech at the conference?'

'Yes, didn't I say?' Derek replies instead of Nick. 'Hers will be on just before yours. She'll be looking at the legal side of wellness and our responsibilities as employers and how we can help our staff. It'll be fascinating, Tara. Can't wait.'

'And,' adds Nick, 'it will certainly help us to try and decide between the two of you. Your qualities as COO are so well matched! It's impossible to choose! But your performances at the conference will certainly make that job easier. Just so you know, Derek and I will be informing you at the end of the conference which one of you has earned the promotion. Something to look forward to, eh? May the best lady win!'

Oh, do fuck off, Nick.

Tara looks smug. I feel sick.

Everything. EVERYTHING is riding on this conference.

Fuck. My. Life.

So, it's later that week on a Thursday night and I'm on the sofa with my laptop. It's not just any old Thursday night. It's the night before . . . not Christmas, but the conference. I'm going through my speech for tomorrow. It's great. I've been working on it for months. It's snappy and witty and informative and interesting. It's taken all the good stuff from my wellness bootcamp experience and showcased how small changes in your life can be very effective. It's even got a tiny bit of harmless mockery of some of the excesses of the wellness industry, so our staff don't think I've gone completely cuckoo. It's sitting there, saved on my laptop, in all its PowerPoint glory (no WordArt, don't worry. I'm not that out of touch). But . . . it's all bollocks really. And especially when it comes to what I say about Clio, what I must say about Clio, because she's our keynote speaker and my speech is on after hers (Tara's is – apparently – just after Clio's, then it's me) and I've been specifically told by Derek to thank her and sing her praises. My God, he's really drunk the Kool-Aid too. And the shittiest thing about it all is that I miss Clio. I actually do. I felt like this really good thing had come into my life after such a long time of feeling totally alone and a bit bleak about everything. And now it turns out this really good thing was all fake. I'm utterly convinced of that now. I can't stop thinking about it. I told Jacqui all about every word of our meeting and she's convinced too. But her research has hit a dead end with the brothers and other aspects of Clio's past. Also she's tried to contact the charities again and they're both saying they're still looking into it. So there's no more news on Clio and no definitive proof she's a liar. It's infuriating. I'm sitting here, the night before the conference when I should be preparing, and all I can do is think about once and for all proving this woman is a fake, this woman I held in such high regard, this woman I foolishly miss from my life.

So I google her website and click on it, just to see her stupid face and remind myself why I shouldn't be missing this scammer at all. And also I'm wondering if those charities are still on her website, after I asked her about them the other week. Yep, they're still there. I hope Jacqui gets some more info on them. Proof from them that they've received nothing would be damning, it really would. But then – hang on – there's something new on her website. There's a new tab called Blog. She didn't keep a blog before. Let's have a look.

Oh. My. Fucking. God.

Clio has started a new blog called – get this – *My Cancer Rematch: How I'm Coping with the Return of my Cancer.*

Let's see what she has to say.

> *Dear Friends,*
> *This is my first ever blog post! I'm always late to the party. I felt it was time to share something with you all. It's not great news, I'm afraid. As you all know, I suffered from cancer several years ago and I recovered and went into remission. I'm sorry to tell you this but the cancer has unfortunately returned. I'm going to be having surgery in a couple of weeks and until then I've been having to go through a number of tests at the hospital. I'm being supported by my friends who have been champions. It's hard to fight this battle alone. That's why I've decided to share my cancer rematch with you: yes, I'm calling it a rematch because I am totally up for this fight. There's no way in heaven or earth that this cancer is going to beat me a second time. The first time I fought back by taking charge of my body and everything that went into it. I refused chemo and went into remission with nutrition. However, this time, there is surgery required to remove a tumour. I embrace wellness in all parts of my life and that includes*

the medical establishment when they can provide skills that I don't have myself, such as surgery. Thank the stars for surgeons and their staff when we really need them. I have the utmost respect for them. However, during my recovery from surgery, I will be instituting my nutritional approach to my body's wellness in order to avoid further need for invasive therapies, such as radio/ chemo. I know that with my gentle weaponry of care for my own body and your support, I will beat back this invader once again. There will always be doubters and nay-sayers who deny the effectiveness of my treatments and question my validity as a therapist, healer and even as a person. You know who you are. And I want to say to you that your lack of support is like a fly on a horse's flank to me. Your negativity is of no consequence to me and will be fought back by me at every step. You have no effect on my wellbeing and you never will. For I know I am surrounded by love and positivity. I have already received wonderful offers of support from many of you reading this now. Thank you for your unending amity, my friends. I am sorry that I will have to stop my therapy sessions for a number of weeks. Many of you already know that and have sent incredible messages of love to keep me afloat in these rough seas. Together we will weather this storm and, never fear, blue skies are ahead. Signing off now to get some rest, until next time, your friend, Clio.

Wow.
Well, I reckon there was a direct threat in there to me. It must be. Unless someone else has started asking questions

as well as me. Below that sanctimonious drivel is a slew of comments from her so-called friends (though they're clearly clients, as many of them mention their therapy and are fangirling).

Warrior woman, you will face this foe and kick its ass! Will miss you and our therapy!

Love u Clio u wonderwoman keep smiling always we hear for u

Oh no Clio I cant believe it dont know what I'll do without our sessions I'm so sorry sending all the good vibes hun

You are a force of nature gorgeous. Don't lose faith. See you back fit and healthy when you're better.

Etc. etc. etc.

And then, underneath all that, is a selfie of Clio, lying in a hospital bed with a drip taped to her hand, looking pale and wan, smiling weakly. Beside her on a side table there are tubes, syringes and medication bottles. Everything looks legit. Her hair looks the same as it did the last time I saw her, so it seems like a recent picture. I stare at it for a while. It looks real. What's going on? I was absolutely certain about her faking cancer. But here she is, large as life, in a hospital bed with a drip. That doesn't happen by chance. Maybe she really is ill. Oh my God, maybe I've got it all wrong . . .

Then I remember what I researched about cancer scammers, about how they get themselves admitted to A&E

and take photos. Could it be that? What about the drip though? You wouldn't get that for nothing. It's in her right hand, taped to it, and the tube runs out of shot, so you can't see the drip itself. That's odd, I mean, if it was legit, wouldn't the drip stand be right next to the bed? I zoom in on her hand and it looks like a drip port should look. I zoom in on other parts of the photo, looking at the medical paraphernalia on the bedside table. I take a good look at every inch of that stuff on the table. The medication bottles – four of them altogether – have labels and I zoom in even further to try to see what's written on them, but they are all turned away from the camera, one on its side again with the label hidden. I look at the tubes and syringes. They're all in packets, brand-new, sitting there. Why are they sitting there? I try to look at the bedstead that she's on. I can't see it because there are white pillows behind her covering it up. I know what the headrests of hospital beds look like and this one is hidden. I can't see it. So I zoom in further to see if there's a hint of it behind those pillows. And I see the white wall behind her. I zoom in further, because I can see now that the wall behind her bed has a kind of texture to it, like Artex or something similar. And once I'm really close I think . . . well, that wall looks like . . . a sheet. Like a flannel sheet. I recognise that kind of weave flannel sheets have as my grandma had them at her house when I was a child and I loved staying there and sleeping in that bed as it had the softest sheets. The wall behind Clio really REALLY looks like it has a flannel sheet hanging behind it and not a wall. What the . . . fuck . . . ? Hang on. I shift over a bit to the side of the photo. Behind the bedside table, right on the left-hand edge of the image, there's a strip of grey. I thought it was the edge of a door frame at first but on closer inspection, it isn't a frame. It's . . . bumpy. And uneven. And that grey is the colour of . . . stone. OH MY GOD!!! It's the unrendered stone from Clio's house!! I know it is!! I've seen it a few times now and there's no doubt in my mind! It's only a strip on the image but it's unmistakable. I can see the separate slabs of rock and the dark dips between them. Oh Clio – I mean oh Julia D-V – how careless of you! How absolutely fucking deliciously stupid of you to fake a hospital picture in your own house and go to the trouble of ordering all that medical equipment off Amazon or wherever and put up a white flannel sheet to double as a hospital ward wall and then not quite crop your photo properly and leave your fucking wall in the shot, you IDIOT! Oh wow, this is it. This is my definitive proof. She's not in the hospital. She's a total fucking liar. She's done this blog to bolster the lie she told me in a panic when I got too close to the truth. Jeez, the desperation of it. It's sickening! Look at you, lady, with your fake pale face. I bet that's make-up! My God, the lengths these scammers will go to. No wonder all the medication bottles are turned away from the camera so we can't see the labels. They're just props! It's all props and fakery!

I've got to tell Jacqui immediately! I go on Clio's website on my phone and screenshot the picture and message it to Jacqui. I'm just about to type an explanation of what it is – plus many, many swear words and exclamation marks – when my phone starts ringing. 'Who the fuck is that?' I cry, as usual. And it turns out, it's Jacqui!

'I was literally just messaging you!' I say, delighted.

'Oh my God, synchronicity or what! I've got dirt, dirt, dirt to dish for you!'

'Me too!!'

'What??'

'No, you go first. What's the dirt?'

I can hear Jacqui take a deep breath.

'Okay . . . prepare yourself. There's good and bad news, kind of.'

'Bad news first. Always.'

'Agreed. Okay, so the charities. I got back to them both this morning and asked to speak to someone more senior and finally got a call back from one of them this evening. So . . . it turns out that there had been no donations from Clio at all since the fundraiser years ago BUT a week ago, Clio sent a donation, suddenly, out of the blue.'

'Oh fucking hell! That's because I bloody mentioned the charities to her! I wish I'd kept my mouth shut about that now. I've been a fool!'

'Don't beat yourself up about it. It's still dodgy. And I've not heard back from the other one yet. Who knows how much money she's pocketed over the years that's not gone in that donation. It definitely needs further investigation.'

'Well, okay. At least it's obvious to us that she's only made that donation because she suddenly had to. Is that the bad news?'

'Yeah, as I said, only kinda bad news. The other news is a doozy. Ready?'

'Yes, yes! Get on with it, woman! I've got the fucking conference tomorrow and I'm shitting myself about all this.'

'Okay, here we go. That little gem you told me about Clio being a chartered surveyor in her past . . . well, I checked that out. And it led me down the garden path, let me tell you. But eventually, today, I found an absolute cracker. So, Clio, under another name of Julie Vincent – basically a slight bastardisation of her real name – Clio and her brother Julian Vincent (I'm guessing that's not his whole name either) had a chartered surveyor business in Hampshire and . . . guess what? The brother Julian was convicted of fraud for writing fake surveys of houses to sell them at a profit! He was jailed for sixty-four months back in 2020, then another case was made two years ago and he's had extra time added to his sentence. It was never proven in court that Clio was involved but she was working shoulder to shoulder with him and I spoke to the local reporter who covered it in Hants and he said he was sure she was involved but the court just couldn't prove it. So, she's definitely been engaged in fraudulent activity before. Or at the very least, very close to it!'

'Oh, fuck me, Jacqui, that's brilliant investigative reporting there! The scammy bitch!'

'Right?! I'm dead proud of myself!'

'You've really knocked it out of the park, Jac. Both of us have, I'd say. We've got the better of that bloody liar, which is quite the feat, considering how good she is at lying. There's just one thing I don't get. Why did she tell different stories to different people when she knew her clients would mix and probably talk about her? I just don't get it.'

'Well,' says Jacqui, 'I reckon it's a case of telling people what they want to hear. And it's good for us to remember that nobody is a criminal mastermind like we see in the movies. People fuck up. Especially when hubris comes into it. They just lie and lie and lie and get the lies mixed up and it all comes crashing down. I've seen that pattern a lot with scammers and criminals I've reported on. They just think they're cleverer than everyone and that they'll never get caught. Until they do.'

'That makes sense, actually. I definitely get the sense she

thought she was better than everyone, now I think of her sitting on that damn podium at the retreat looking like the Queen of fucking Sheba.'

'Urgh! Hateful. But listen, what have you found out?'

I tell Jacqui all about the picture I've just sent. She has a look at it and I point out all the fakery and the wall and she can see it too.

'It's definitely a stone wall!' cries Jacqui. 'I've never even been to her house and I can see that. Oh Clio, how clumsy of you, my dear!'

'I know! It's hilarious!'

'Wow, she's really getting desperate now. Faking cancer again and starting a blog, after all these years of anonymity on social media. She's running scared. She knows you're onto her and is ramping up, not backing down. What the hell are you going to do about the conference tomorrow?'

I feel a nauseous lurch in my stomach. Back to reality.

'Oh God, I don't know. I'm wracking my brains about it. Tara hasn't said a word to me since our massive fallout. Derek and Nick think Clio is the dog's bollocks. And I know in my heart she's a total faker. But this conference is going to be the decider on who gets the promotion, me or Tara. And if I call out Clio now, it'll go down like a sack of shit for me. It'll blow the promotion, no doubt in my mind. It's all . . . too much to figure out. God knows what I'm going to do. I need to think. I'll message you later. I'll let you know what I decide. Fuck, it's half seven. The evening is ebbing away. I need to get on with finishing my speech now.'

'Okay, chick. Listen, call me if you need to, okay?'

'I will, thanks, darling. And thank you for that news. You are amazing!'

'Oh pish-tish. Talk soon. Bye.'

'Bye, love.'

So, my situation is as follows. I have set up Clio as a guru at the staff conference but now I know that Clio is a fraud, I'll have to bite the bullet and tell my boss, the old CEO, Derek. What will Nick, the new CEO, think of my tremendous gaffe? My chances for promotion will be toast. I briefly consider letting the whole thing slide and just letting Clio do her speech and keeping quiet. But what if she scams people at work afterwards, just like she scammed me? You know what, I've realised something. I know of five separate people at work who've had cancer and gone into remission. And three more with spouses who've had cancer. This is the other side of being director of HR: it's not all telling people off for having the word MOTHERFUCKER emblazoned on a mug. You get to see people at their lowest and you help them through it, you make sure that their experience in the work environment helps them rather than hinders them. You show some bloody empathy and you help them get back to work when they're ready and only when they're ready. We did it through the pandemic and we're still doing it now: every day, someone needs you in HR. Someone's ill and needs your support. And if I let Clio Kenton stand up there and blather on about her fake cancer and sway some of my staff – MY staff, yes! They are mine! They're like my extended family, for heaven's sake, as much as I moan about them . . . I don't want a single one of them falling for Clio's bullshit and giving her their hard-earned money to scam them about drinking mango juice to cure their cancer or whatever the fuck. It's actually made me realise that I really do care about the people at work; I don't want any of them – even the arseholes! – to become Clio's next prey. Plus, once this fraud business comes out – which with Jacqui's investigating, even if she doesn't get the article in the paper, just the questions she's asking will probably stir things up enough for other people to ask questions too and start digging, especially those charities – once the news is out that Clio is full of shit, I'll be ruined at work anyway. There's nothing else for it. I know what I have to do now.

I get up from the sofa, get my shoes and my jacket on, grab my car keys and head out of my house.

Chapter 26

The front door opens. It's Janey, Derek's wife. It's 8pm and she's probably wondering what the hell her husband's director of HR is doing ringing her doorbell after hours, like some kind of bad movie.

'Lucy! Is . . . everything all right?'

Janey is so nice. She doesn't deserve a wanker of a husband. About this time of night at home I'd be in pyjamas and slippers but she's fully dressed in smart beige slacks and a silky cream shirt with perfectly coiffed dark grey hair pulled back into a neat bun at her neck. She's a woman who has a wealthy husband and has never needed to work, but I do know she volunteers at a range of organisations and charities, to help other people. And I bloody applaud her for that. She works hard for no pay just because she can and that's admirable. Not like her polar opposite, Clio.

'Janey, I'm so sorry to bother you both at night. I know it's madly unorthodox.'

'No problem at all, love. Come in out of the cold. We had

a sort of false spring last week, didn't we, but this week it's all frosty mornings and chilly nights again.'

Nice, you see? So nice. I step in over the threshold and stand in their hall, which has a side table for letters, keys and a phone, as well as a hat stand and umbrella stand. It's delightfully old-fashioned and I love it. I feel like I'm visiting my grandparents' house, even though there's probably only fifteen years or so between us. Janey shuts the front door.

'Would you like a warming drink? Tea, coffee, Ovaltine?'

God, what I wouldn't give to have a mug of Ovaltine with Janey right now and just sit on her sofa and tell her all my woes. But I can't. I'm not there to see her, more's the pity.

'I won't, thanks, Janey. I really need to see Derek, if possible. It's quite urgent.'

'Of course. He's upstairs in his study. I'll fetch him. He always says he has various work things to be doing up there but I know he's actually playing Wordle because I just spied it on his monitor through the door.'

'Thank you,' I say, chuckling at the thought of Derek being addicted to Wordle. I mean, I am too – I play it every night in bed before I go to sleep – but I didn't put Derek down as a Wordle man. People can be so different outside of work to how you'd imagine them to be.

Janey shows me into their front room and I sit down on the sofa and wait. It's a lovely room, filled with classy knick-knacks, like antique photo frames and little china figures, local glossy magazines on the coffee table, *The Telegraph* and *The Times* beside it, and lamps with a warm glow spilling across the thick, soft carpets. Yet, despite the charming milieu, I feel sick, really sick. I don't know what the outcome of this meeting is going to be but I know it's going to be bad, either

297

way. There is no positive outcome to this for me. But there could be for others and that's who I need to focus on now: Clio's future victims.

I hear a few muffled words being had upstairs and then the sound of creaking footsteps on the staircase. And then Derek is coming through the door. He's in a maroon dressing gown, tartan flannel pyjamas and leather slippers, yet he holds his dignity even in that get-up. And I feel rotten for intruding on him like this and not calling first. But I couldn't risk him not answering or putting me off. This needs to be done face to face.

'Why, Lucia!' he says, his voice as loud and strident at home as in the office. Some things don't change.

I stand up to greet him. 'Derek, I must apologise for this unprecedented visit. I wouldn't have come so late if it wasn't of the utmost importance.'

'It's not a problem, Lucia. Please take a seat and tell me what this is all about. I have no doubt we can sort it easily.'

I wish I had his blind confidence. He sits down opposite me in an armchair, legs crossed, looking completely at ease despite being caught in his pyjamas at night. I begrudgingly admire him for that and for not betraying any annoyance at my intrusion.

'Thank you for seeing me. So, I have some information about our keynote speaker – Clio Kenton – that I feel I must share with you. In fact, I feel it is my duty to share with you.'

Derek's face betrays nothing. He says simply, 'Go on.'

'Well . . . it's come to my attention that Clio Kenton isn't all that she seems to be. In fact, I have significant doubts of her qualifications to practise the work that she does and also there may well be an illegal aspect to her profession, though I don't have solid proof for this as yet.'

Derek sits up now and leans forward. 'Go on,' he says again, a man of few words when it comes to serious matters.

And so I begin. I tell him everything I know about Clio Kenton, in the order I discovered it. I tell him about Jacqui and her investigative research. I tell him how sorry I am that I didn't do this kind of research myself before I introduced Clio into our business and that I take full responsibility for it. I finish by stating my conclusion to this sorry state of affairs:

'If at all possible, I believe we should withdraw Clio Kenton as keynote speaker for tomorrow's event and yet it's likely we'll still need to pay her fee, for which again I can only apologise. I felt it necessary to bring all of this to your attention tonight and again I'm only sorry I wasn't able to bring this to you earlier, yet the final nail in the coffin for me was hearing that her family member had been imprisoned for fraud in a business she was so closely involved in. That's when I knew that it was time to discuss it with you. In my view, we need to cancel her speech tomorrow and remove all mention of her from everyone else's speeches and materials.'

There's a long pause while Derek considers all of this. He's been listening intently to every word I've said, without taking his gaze off me. Now he sits back in his chair and links his hands together and rests his chin on them, a picture of contemplation. I've really no idea what he's going to say next.

'That's not going to happen, I'm afraid, Lucia.'

'I'm sorry?'

'I dare say you should be. Coming here, unannounced, on the night before the conference, with a web of unconfirmed chitter-chatter about our star speaker?'

I'm surprised at that. Derek usually has faith in me to do

my job properly. As annoying as he is, he's never doubted my judgement.

'Erm . . . well . . . I know it's unconfirmed. But I believe the evidence is piling up against Clio Kenton. I believe it is persuasive and certainly warrants further investigation before allowing her to represent us and our wellness strategy to our employees. If it does turn out that her practice is fraudulent, then this will reflect very badly on our management of the company.'

'And that's why we won't be doing a thing. You could've come to me weeks ago, by the sounds of it, with your concerns. But you didn't. You've left it to the very last minute. And what you don't know is that Clio Kenton is not only delivering our keynote speech but also, unbeknownst to you or anyone else in the company except Nick Bridges, we've also signed a contract with Clio to become a freelance executive staff member, as director of workplace wellbeing, and on a hefty fee, I may add. We plan to announce it tomorrow, at the conference. All of our printed materials that Nick Bridges has had produced and will distribute tomorrow have this information in. My speech and Nick's both talk about Clio too. And Tara's, no doubt. Clio is integral to our new wellness policy and the lynchpin of the entire conference.'

I'm flabbergasted. I cannot believe this is happening. I'm also raging. How dare the CEOs appoint a new member of staff without any oversight from me!

'As director of HR, I'm amazed you thought it wise to hand out a senior role at Beane & Co to a freelancer without doing the proper checks and without first consulting me! You've gone completely over my head!'

Derek looks mad now. 'Because that's what CEOs do. They

act decisively. We don't need to come running to a woman for permission to do our damned jobs!'

Oh, I see now. To a *woman*. Or to this woman in particular, to me. Christ, I thought I could appeal to his better nature. But the longer I know Derek, the more I doubt he has one, even if he is a fellow Wordle fan.

'Derek, if this comes out after tomorrow, that Clio Kenton is indeed a fraud, then her involvement in our company could be catastrophic for our public image. It'll be a dreadful embarrassment for Beane & Co. Customers could desert us in droves.'

'Well, it's not going to come out, even if there is anything there.'

I'm confused. What's he saying?

He goes on, 'Because you're going to keep everything you've told me under wraps. And you're going to tell that journalist friend of yours to shelve it, as well. Because if you want this promotion, and this ever comes out about Clio Kenton, especially now she's so intimately involved in our company, then your career will be in tatters. And there's something else you don't know and that is about Janey.'

Derek stops here and runs his fingers through his hair and sighs.

'What . . . what about Janey?'

Derek looks up at me, defiantly. 'Janey has ovarian cancer. She's starting treatment soon. When you first told me about Clio, I told Janey and now Janey's been seeing Clio for a few weeks and the change in her has been tremendous. She's come from despair to hope for the first time in a long time. Clio is an integral part of her recovery programme. She's written a treatment plan for Janey that's going to help her immeasurably. Clio Kenton has saved us in ways you can't even imagine, so I don't want to hear any more of your nasty little nuggets of gossip.'

Oh God, Janey. Not Janey too. This is horrible. Clio attracts these poor people with cancer like a magnet. I can't let this happen.

'Derek, I am telling you in the strongest terms possible. You must get Janey away from Clio Kenton, as far away from her influence as you can. Clio did not cure herself with nutrition or anything else. I strongly believe that she never had cancer in the first place. This is dangerous stuff, Derek. This isn't just about the business. I'm not exaggerating. This is life and death for Janey.'

Derek stands up and shouts at me, 'How dare you come here and mention that word and my wife's name in the same sentence!'

He's visibly shaking now. Oh Christ, this has descended into a nightmare. I stand up and pick up my handbag. It's clear I mustn't stay here a moment longer. Nothing I say will make any difference. He's sold, long gone, drunk the Kool-Aid and gone back for seconds and thirds. And so has his lovely wife.

'I am sorry,' I say, looking at the floor, to give him time to recover himself. 'I'll go now. Apologies again for my intrusion.'

I look up and Derek is standing with his hands thrust in his dressing gown pockets, his chin jutting out in proud defiance.

'I should think so too. The conference will go ahead as planned tomorrow. These unfounded claims you will shelve and keep to yourself. I can only imagine it's envy of Clio's skills and position that has driven you. It doesn't look good for you, Lucia. But to be as fair as I can, I will not be mentioning this to anyone and certainly not to Nick Bridges. If you deliver your speech at the conference as planned and otherwise keep your head down, you're still in the running for COO. But any suggestion that you wish to sabotage the conference or Clio Kenton's work at Beane & Co or – and let me make this very clear – any attempt to interfere in Clio's place in my personal life and that of my wife, will result in my very strong objection to Nick that the COO post should not under any circumstances be yours. And believe me, Nick Bridges listens to every word I say and will do what I advise, be certain of that. And with that, I think you should leave now, Lucia. I shall see you at the conference bright and early tomorrow. You can see yourself out.'

I nod and leave the room. As I go into the hallway, I see Janey coming down the stairs. She hasn't seen me yet. I could stay, I could tell her to beware Clio, to never go back, never listen to another lying word that fraudster says. But then Derek appears in the doorway, watching me like a hawk. Janey comes to the bottom of the stairs and I can tell she's about to say something nice, as ever, her sweet smile on her face.

I swiftly turn and leave the hallway, pulling the front door closed behind me.

I can only hope that Derek calms down, thinks again about what I've told him and – even if the conference goes ahead as planned – does some sniffing around himself about the person whose hands he's putting his wife's life into. I can but hope. I feel like the worst coward in the world for not shouting something out to Janey. But I couldn't, I just couldn't.

Chapter 27

I feel like I'm crawling away to my car, like some craven animal. I should've stood up to Derek, I should've resigned. But the promotion . . . the COO post . . . I've wanted it for so long. I've worked myself to death for it. I can't give it up now. I simply can't.

And now I have to swallow it all and give my speech as if nothing has happened. And I have to tell Jacqui to shelve that article and never speak of it again. That article that could help her career. That should be written. That should be out there, helping other people, getting justice for the many Clio has lied to and is still lying to, who spend their money on her, who donate to charities she rarely pays, who put their cancer treatment into her care, her fraudulent, lying care, to their own detriment, maybe even to the demise of their own health, or even lead to their own . . . death. It is *that* bad.

I'm in my car driving home. I know what I must do now. I pull over at the side of the road. I go on WhatsApp and I make a call. It rings and rings. Finally, someone answers.

'Lucy?' says Tara, in a snippy voice. We've not spoken since our falling-out. She's barely even looked at me since then.

'Tara, thanks for answering.'

'Of course. It is about work, I'm assuming?'

'Yes,' I say, feeling miserable. But I must go on. I tell her everything that just happened. I tell her about Janey and her cancer, about Derek's position. I wait to hear what she has to say.

'I don't know what you think you want from me,' replies Tara, curtly. 'I'm one hundred per cent on Derek's side. Honestly, Lucy, this kind of behaviour is erratic. Not what I'd expect from an HR director. Driving around at night hurling accusations about. Your so-called evidence against Clio is all hearsay. There's nothing concrete there at all. Legally, you're on very thin ice with all this. If Clio were told you're going around saying these things about her, she'd be quite within her rights to sue you for slander. That's what I would do if I were her.'

Jesus, that's low. And it sounds like a threat, that Tara might tell Clio what I've been saying. But it also shows me that Tara is completely fooled by her too. And defensive. Nobody wants to admit they've been duped. Derek, Tara – they both hate the idea that, as mature, experienced and intelligent people of standing in the community, they've been taken for a ride. They can't bear it. They have to deny it, because allowing the possibility of it is an admission of their own weakness. And neither of them can tolerate that.

'Okay, Tara,' I say, my temples pounding now with a stress headache. 'I'm going now. I won't bother you again. I just ask one thing. Go and look at Clio's website. Look at that hospital bed picture. Look at the left-hand side. And ask yourself, categorically – is that a hospital ward wall, or is it a white flannel sheet hung up on Clio's unrendered stone walls at home? And if so, why the hell is she taking fake hospital selfies if she really has cancer, if she really ever had it at all? Just go and look at that picture. That's all I ask.'

Then, I ring off. I finish my drive home and collapse on the sofa. I don't know what to do. I consider my options. I could resign tonight and forfeit years of struggle to get that COO post. But if I resign, my staff will be subjected to the bullshit of Clio Kenton and there will be nobody there to protect them from it. I could go to the conference and tell them the truth, stand up there and publicly denounce Clio and risk being sued for slander because I don't have any proper proof whatsoever, just hearsay and circumstantial evidence and a gut feeling. Is that enough to ruin my career and risk legal action? Or I could not resign and go to the conference tomorrow and deliver my speech and not rock the boat, swallow everything and be in with a chance of getting my promotion. If I do that, I need to ring Jacqui, tell her to shelve her research and pretend all of this never happened, so that I can keep my job. Would she do that for me? She probably would. She said she would. She said she'd stop if I asked her to. So I could ask her. And everything would go back to normal. And work would be fine. And I'd be back in the running for my dream job.

I pick up my phone. I'm going to call Jacqui and ask her to keep it all quiet. But I feel physically and mentally wretched about it. How can I do that to Jacqui, take away this great story from her that might help her career? Also, how can I look my dear friend in the face again if I've knowingly allowed a scammer to be let loose on vulnerable people and forced my best friend to do the same, for my own personal gain? I can't believe how far I've sunk. I used to have principles, things I believed in, about protecting my staff and encouraging honest and open work practices. Now I'm going to be a liar, lying to my staff, telling them wellness bullshit to please my boss, unleashing Clio Kenton on their unsuspecting lives. I'll be a liar for my own profit. I'll be a scammer, just like Clio.

And I can't do that.

I think about calling Jacqui and asking her advice. But you know what, she has enough on her plate. Harvey is having a blood test done tomorrow morning, when I'm giving the speech. I'd asked Jacqui if she'd come, for moral support. She's not on the staff, obviously, but being director of HR has its privileges and nobody would question it if I had a friend there. But she said she couldn't, as she'd be taking Harvey to the hospital for yet another blood test requested by his GP, who is still refusing to refer him to a rheumatologist after Jacqui asking a dozen times. God, I wish she'd let me pay for a private specialist. I know what I'll do. I have her bank account details. Sometimes we pay for stuff for each other then forward the money back. I go on my banking app and I send her a thousand pounds from my savings. That should cover at least two or three appointments or so with a private specialist. I'm hoping she could get to see someone privately and then they'd send Harvey for any tests via the NHS so they could get it without having to pay. But either way, I'll make sure she has enough money to cover it. There's no way I'm going to stand by and watch her lad suffer like this. That's sorted then. Now, to work.

I grab my laptop and open it up, pulling up my PowerPoint presentation. I fetch a bottle of Turkish wine, the splendid

Buzbag Reserve. I get on my phone and order a Turkish takeaway to go with it: a lamb shish with chargrilled aubergine and garlic. I start retyping my presentation. I'm ditching almost everything I've written so far and putting in new material. My fingers are flying now. My mind is on fire. It takes me hours, but I've finally finished it. I read it through. I imagine saying all of this tomorrow and I feel shaky at the thought of it. It's a total takedown of Clio Kenton. All the facts, all the hunches, all the hearsay that damns her. I know it's not legally sound but I don't care. I'm not going to let this scammy liar loose on my staff. It'll be a disaster for the company. I know delivering this speech will ruin everything for me. But I don't care. Janey always comes to the staff conference and she'll hear it too. I have to do it, for her, for my staff, for everyone. The world needs to know that Clio Kenton is a fraud.

It's sitting there on my laptop, done. I'm trembling. Can I really do it, read that out tomorrow to hundreds of people, with Clio Kenton – the accused – watching me? What will happen? Will Clio cry and pretend to faint? Will Derek throw a chair at me? Would Nick Bridges manhandle me off the stage? My God, it could descend into farce.

I'm scared. I don't know if I can do it. I pick up my plate with a bit of delectable lamb left on it and I finish it off, for strength. I upend my glass of Buzbag and finish that off too, for fortitude. Then I look at the time. It's nearly midnight. I feel very alone in this. I admit to myself that I'm terrified.

Then my phone bleeps a message. Who can that be at this time? I have a look. It's a meme from Noah, my nearly fifteen-year-old nephew in New Zealand. It's a drawing of a little man standing next to a pond, looking down at a fish that's popped up out of the water to look around. The man says, 'Are you the legendary talking fish?' And the fish says, 'No.'

I laugh aloud. Noah always sends me the funniest shit. I message back.

That's ace. What are you up to? Aren't you supposed to be learning useless information – about vectors and algebra that you'll never once use again in your life – at school right now?

New Zealand is thirteen hours ahead, so it'll be lunchtime there about now. Maybe he's in the school yard or the lunch room, eating whatever Kiwis eat for lunch. He's a lucky lad. My sister and her husband have given them a lovely life over there, they really have.

But there's no reply. There very rarely is from Noah. He just sends me funny stuff and I reply and he's already moved on to other things in his busy teenage life. But I appreciate the random thought. I appreciate it hugely. My nephew could easily have forgotten his rather useless aunt thousands of miles away and six years since I've seen him in real life, since he was eight years old. I find it incredibly touching that he still reaches out across the ocean with hilarious little jokes to connect with me.

God, I feel so alone right now. With the shitshow of tomorrow approaching fast, this really feels like my dark night of the soul. It's really late. I can't call Jacqui for support. She'll be asleep and she really needs her sleep with her job and home and the kids and everything she does for them. It's gone midnight here now, approaching 1am. But . . . hang on . . . in New Zealand of course, it isn't night. Maybe Shirl and Mum will be home. Maybe they'll be having a sandwich. Maybe I could say hi. I think I'd feel grounded if I could see their faces.

I message Shirley.

Shirl, could I video call with you guys? Like, right now? If you're free. I know it sounds silly. I'm just struggling with something. And I'd really like to see you, and Mum. All of you, if anyone else is there, though I guess the boys are at school and Ray is at work. I just miss you all, that's all. Sorry if this sounds daft.

I wait.

I've been so neglectful of them. Why would they be there for me in my time of need? I sink down into the sofa. This is what happens when you devote your life to one thing to the detriment of others. You end up alone, on the sofa, past midnight, with nobody to talk to. God, I feel low.

Then my phone chimes. I grab it.

OK. Kids are here actually. Baker day at school. We're having a barbecue & Ray got the day off. Good timing. Hang on.

You're always having barbecues! You're such a cliché of Brits in the antipodes!

I feel excited. And nervous. I don't know why I feel nervous. It's my family. But . . . I never do things like this. I so often feel like communicating with my family is a chore. But right now, I want it more than anything in the world.

My phone rings and I tap on the camera.

The first thing I see is a big bowl of potato salad. Oh. My. God. Mum always used to make the BEST potato salad. She'd use Charlotte potatoes and homemade mayo and put in chives and mustard and God knows what else, but it always tasted amazing. Then I see Shirl's face.

'Did Mum make that?!' I ask.

'She sure did. It's your favourite. You always used to have orgasms over it.'

'Muuu-uuum!!!' cries a voice off. 'You can't go around saying orgasms willy-nilly!'

It's Noah, my older nephew. I'd recognise that sarcastic voice with great vocabulary anywhere.

'What's a willy-nilly?' says another voice in the background.

That's Ned, my younger nephew. I don't know him so well. He doesn't have a phone yet. My sister won't allow it until he's thirteen, for some arbitrary reason. But I can understand why. She's terrified about online porn and addictive social media ruining her boys' brains. So I don't get memes from Ned. He's much quieter than Noah, an introvert. He likes science and bugs. I'd like to talk about bugs with him. I'd like to get to know that interesting mind he has, that he keeps closely guarded, behind his shyness. But it's almost impossible to do that, when you're on the other side of the planet.

'Hey, lads! Show your faces then!' I cry.

Shirl turns the phone around and I see the two boys in their garden, the sun bright, the foliage lime green behind them. They're chomping down on hotdogs with piles of onions by the looks of it, as Ned's onions are dropping off his hotdog onto the grass every time he takes a bite. They're busy with food, I can see. They wave and manage to shout Hey and Hi with their mouths full.

Then I get a quick view of Ray, the dentist, the nice guy, dressed in stripy T-shirt and shorts, his tummy sticking out, his short hair greying and neatly combed, who's always supported Shirl in everything she's done and is a great dad to those boys. He waves his tongs and says, 'All right, Lucy!' Then returns to lovingly tending his sizzling slabs of meat.

The phone goes back to Shirl's face.

'You all right?' she says in a businesslike way, doing her duty.

'Not really,' I say. 'Just some work stuff.'

It's a massive understatement. But I don't even know how to start explaining it all to my sister, especially not while she's having yet another nice sunny barbecue with her family.

Shirl rolls her eyes. 'Always with the work stuff.'

I know why she's bitter about it. She thinks I chose my job over my family. And she's not wrong. I did. I felt my choice was justified. I still think that. But I know now I sacrificed certain aspects of my life. And tonight, for the first time in years, I'm actually questioning . . . was it worth it?

'Mum's here,' adds Shirl. 'Want to see her?'

'Absolutely,' I say. God, I think I'm going to cry. I must contain myself. I can't ruin their bright New Zealand day with my problems.

Then I see Mum, sitting at a garden table, fork in hand, eating her delicious potato salad. She waves at the camera and I wave back. She looks so old, she looks more frail than when I saw her on the last video call. She looks small. And far away.

Then she puts her fork down and waves at Shirley with

her mouth full, gesturing for the phone. She finishes off her chewing and looks into the camera, holding the phone now.

'What's up, Lu-Lu?' she says.

It still affects me, hearing her call me that, Dad's nickname for me. I really am going to start bawling in a minute. I force myself not to cry.

'Just some crappy stuff at work, Mum. Nothing to worry about.'

'But I am worried. You don't call Shirl unless something's wrong, most of the time.'

Then I feel guilty about that. That I only get in touch with my sister when I need something. That really is shitty.

'I'm sorry, Mum. I'm sorry about that.'

She looks confused.

'What are you sorry about now?'

'I don't know, Mum. Just everything. I'm sorry I haven't been out to see you guys. I'm sorry I put work first for so long. I'm sorry I sacrificed everything for this dumb job.'

I haven't spoken like this to Mum in years. I don't know where all this is coming from, but it feels about as stoppable as an avalanche.

'Don't be sorry,' says Mum. 'I'm proud of you.'

Her brown eyes are twinkling as she smiles at the camera.

'Whatever are you proud of *me* for?'

'You're a director in an insurance company. Not even your dad got that far up the ladder. I tell all my friends that. And my hairdresser. And the chiropodist. Everyone's always impressed by that.'

'I'm not sure it means anything anymore, Mum,' I say miserably, fighting back the tears. I really, really don't want to cry in front of her. It's not fair. It's not right that I throw my misery before them like a gauntlet, when I've done so little to help them with their grief over the years they went away. It's just not right.

'But, Mum,' I say, gathering myself. 'I'm okay. I know what I'm going to do about this work problem. I'm going to sort it. It'll be fine.'

'I know you will,' says Mum.

Then she pauses and looks down, then looks up at the camera again.

'Come and see us soon, won't you, Lu?'

'Maybe I will,' I say. I can't take this anymore, my mum's sweet face, calling me Lu when she never did, my sister's happy life. I have to get off this call or I'll blub like a baby. 'Bye, Mum. Say bye to Shirl and Ray and the boys for me. Love you.'

I don't wait for her reply. I tap the red end call symbol and throw the phone down on the sofa and sob. And sob and sob.

What the hell am I going to do? What the hell will happen tomorrow? Can I really do that rewritten speech, that hatchet job on a scammer that will ruin my work life and probably get me sued, all alone, up there on that stage, in front of every single person at work, before the CEOs, and the directors, and the managers, and the staff, and my former guru, the fallen angel, that fraudulent fucker Clio Kenton??

Then, my doorbell goes. I stop crying instantly. Did I really hear that?

Then it goes again. It's definitely my doorbell.

Who in the name of FUCK can that be, at this time of night?!

Chapter 28

The local cinema is a newish one, but not new enough to have those recliner seats and the fancy-shmancy side tables. It's just old enough to have inordinately uncomfortable chairs that feel like they're stuffed with horse hair and give only just enough leg room for a pygmy goat. All of our staff are milling around, in and out of the rows, while they gather around the food tables. We've arranged for the cinema to give everyone pizza slices, loaded wedges, mozzarella sticks and taco chips with dips, with slushies or tea and coffee to drink. It is the annual staff conference, held on a Friday at the end of March, ready for the new tax year. The morning is spent in conference rooms at the office, while we go through separate department meetings and then everyone repairs to the cinema for lunch and the afternoon's conference speeches. After the speeches, everyone tends to hang around as the private bar opens and quite a few people get sloshed. Everyone's in a great mood. There are huge banners everywhere of Clio, presumably done by Nick Bridges. And there Clio is, over by the bar, talking to

Nick and Tara. Clio is preening herself in some very upmarket lilac athleisure wear. Derek's nearby talking away to two of the other directors, his face plastered in smiles, until he spots me across the room and looks daggers at me. *Don't you dare*, his look seems to say. His lovely wife Janey appears from the direction of the loos and comes up beside him and links arms with him. Oh God . . . Janey.

It's just turned 2pm, time for the speeches to begin. Everyone is filing into the auditorium and filling up the seats. I ascend the stairs to the stage and disappear into the wings. My speech isn't quite yet. We've got a few to go first. So I'll have to stand here and sweat buckets while I'm waiting. The room smells of myriad different perfumes and aftershaves, along with old pizza, spicy salsa and the odd whiff of cigarette smoke. What I wouldn't give to deeply inhale a cigarette about now and I don't even smoke anymore. Or sip a measure of Dalmore twelve-year-old single malt whisky. Anything, to take the edge off. My phone vibrates in my pocket. I quickly check it to see it's a message from Jacqui. She's asking why the hell she has a grand in her current account from me. And she says she's crying. The reference I put on the payment was *For Harvey No Return*. I smile to myself. I'll reply later. Hopefully she won't send it back. Hopefully I can send her more when she needs it. And we'll get that boy helped and he'll feel a lot better a lot sooner. I put my phone back in my pocket. It's nearly zero hour. I must focus now.

Derek is up first. His PA Sharon sets up his PowerPoint for him on the vast cinema screen behind him, as well as ensuring his clipped-on microphone works and once that's all done, he brings the crowd to a hush. He speaks in his customarily loud voice, even though he's miked up and the fish that live in unexplored underground caves a mile below the earth's surface could hear him. He does his rather tedious round-up of the past twelve months, prizes are awarded to various members of staff, targets are celebrated and then Derek starts to wax lyrical about his decades at the company, seeing as this is his last ever staff conference. Retirement, endless rounds of golf and warmer climes beckon, he tells everyone. Only a few of us know that he and Janey aren't going anywhere soon, not in Janey's condition. I watch her watching him, from the front row. Her face is glowing. She's so proud of him. Christ, don't cry, I tell myself. You'll make your mascara run. And I'm not nearly crying for Derek's exit, obviously; I'm crying for Janey and that fucking fraud Clio Kenton, sitting to one side of Derek as he makes his speech, beside Nick Bridges who keeps chatting her up. I can't bear to look at them. The room gives Derek a thumping round of applause as he departs, which is strangely touching. He is a pain in the arse, Derek, but we all knew him and could predict him and we've all put up with him for years. Better the devil you know and all that. I find that I'm actually a little sorry to see him go. But only because I've no idea what our next speaker will do when he takes over as CEO. Especially after my performance today . . .

Derek goes to sit down beside Clio. Only the two CEOs and the keynote speaker are seated on the stage. All the other directors are on the front row, along with the odd wife or husband here or there. That's why I'm waiting here in the wings. I don't want to have to trip up the stairs to get to the podium, though I'm that nervous, I'll probably trip up over my feet as I walk over there. Waiting here, I suddenly think back to my first session with Clio, where I was in one of the old musicals I used to watch with Dad. I've not thought about that daydream much since but I think I understand it now. I was waiting in the wings, not wanting to be the performer. But maybe it was about more than that. Maybe it was really about how I've been waiting in the wings of my own life, of my own self, waiting for my life to change, if I got that promotion. Plus it was all about how much I miss Dad, how I can't leave him behind. But . . . maybe I should. Maybe it's time to stop waiting in the wings for my life to get better. Maybe it's time to take centre stage. Whatever else Clio has done, she did give me that . . . which makes her fraudulent acts even more despicable.

Next up on stage is Nick Bridges, our new CEO. His speech is all about looking forward, replete with alpha-male language like things 'forging' and 'thrusting' ahead. Then he shows his softer, more human side and waffles on about the integrity of the company and how lucky he is to be blessed with such a great staff and though there will be a reshuffle, there will be nothing to fear for staff. I wonder if that's bullshit. I wonder if there will be a raft of involuntary redundancies on Monday, starting with my own. I'm watching my staff watch Nick and they are nervous, I can see it in their eyes, their hunched over stances and their whispers to each other. Nobody knows what to expect. I feel protective of them. I hope this CEO doesn't come in and stomp all over them. Oh, I know quite a few of them are petty or lazy or flaky or annoying reprobates, but they're MY reprobates. And I don't want anyone fucking them over. Not on my watch.

Nick brings things to an end with a series of spreadsheets and graphs on his PowerPoint which few of us actually understand and drives everyone to glazed-eyed expressions that may as well be eyes painted on fake glasses for the interest they're showing. Nick doesn't get such a resounding round of applause as Derek did. He looks a bit put out. Then he turns and introduces our star speaker of the conference, the woman nobody could miss plastered on the oversized banners plonked all over the cinema. I feel like I'm being haunted by multiple cardboard Clios, all staring at me murderously. Fucking hell. Here she comes, walking up to the podium, my staff clapping her hesitantly as none of them know who the hell she is. And I wish that's the way it would stay. But of course it won't.

For Clio tells them all her tale of woe. Here she goes again, talking about the many cancers that ate through her poor body. Oh, she's using every kind of rhetorical device to ham up this web of lies: simile, metaphor, rule of three, direct address, etc. etc. etc. She knows her stuff does Clio. She knows how to grab attention and keep it. She knows how to elicit sympathy and twist it until everyone's misty-eyed. I watch my staff from the side of the stage, see them fall under her spell. Women leaning their faces forward and resting their elbows on their knees, chins on hands. Men are not fidgeting or whispering. Everyone is rapt. Listening to every lying word Clio weaves makes me feel sick. I mean, I've felt all morning like I'm going to vomit. I couldn't eat a bit of lunch. I had a crumbly oat energy bar in the car this morning, about as moist as sawdust and couldn't stomach anything but coffee since then. I'm buzzing like a kid fuelled up on Smarties washed down with Coca-Cola. I'm standing at the edge of oblivion, vibrating with caffeine, totally alone before the abyss.

But then, I feel a tap on my shoulder.

I turn around and it's Tara.

'Where the fuck have you been?' I whisper.

'I've had the shits all bloody day.'

'Oh Christ!' I say and slap my hand over my mouth to stop myself giggling. Tara is doing the same. We're shaking our heads and trying not to burst out laughing at a hugely inappropriate moment as Clio continues to throw out lies left, right and centre about her famed cancer treatment programme. 'Do you want some Imodium? I've got some in my bag.'

'No, I've already taken enough to stun a small horse.'

God, I really want to laugh out loud. Thank fuck for Tara.

'Are you definitely up for this?' she says and squeezes my arm.

'I'm champing at the damn bit, lady,' I say.

For the mystery guest who turned up at my house gone midnight last night was . . . Tara Harryman.

She'd spent the whole evening staring at that blog post picture of Clio's. She'd zoomed in on that left-hand edge a hundred times. And she knew, as sure as eggs is eggs, that Clio's hospital selfie was snapped in her barn conversion with the bare stone walls. It took her all evening to decide what to do. And in the end, even though it was the promotion she wanted, she couldn't let me go through it alone. She came round and she read my speech. And she said, in no uncertain terms, 'You can't bloody say all that!' And I knew she was right. But what else could I do? 'I'm the legal expert round here,' she reminded me. 'Let me have a go at it.' And Tara started to rewrite my speech, with me in attendance, slurping Buzbag Reserve and making coffee to keep us awake, while we worked into the early hours, amalgamating our speeches into one great opus together, both of us on fire, both of us throwing in words and phrases and sentences to really make it sing. By 3am we were ready. She drove home, I set my alarm and passed out on the sofa. We were both up at seven, ready for the most important speech of our working lives. Consummate professionals, you see? Turns out we are both the best woman for the job.

And now it's Tara's turn for her speech. She looks at me in the wings, ready to go on. We spontaneously give each other a hug and grasp each other's hands.

'Ready?' she says.

'Fuck yeah,' I say.

And together, we stride over to the podium. Derek's PA Sharon looks confused. She's got Tara's original PowerPoint all ready up on the screen. But Tara tells her not to worry and explains we've got a new one, we're doing our speech together and she'll sort it. Sharon edges off, looking confused. I glance over at Nick Bridges and he looks intrigued. Derek looks suspicious as hell. And Clio . . . oh, her face is my favourite. She looks worried. Really worried. And I look her dead in the eye and smirk at her with triumph. Hold on to your athleisure wear, Clio, you scammy sociopath.

Here we go.

It's time for a take-down.

Chapter 29

We stand together, Tara and I. Tara taps on our joint PowerPoint to start it off. On the screen is a montage of a variety of people, some sitting in yoga poses, some drinking juice cleanses, some caught running away down a street. They are all real-life wellness scammers, from yogic masters accused of fraud, sexual assault and even sex trafficking, to grifter influencers pretending to be sick and touting fake medicines, to Machiavellian gurus defrauding millions out of brainwashed cult followers.

Tara begins.

'What if the most powerful influence in your life – something and someone you deeply believe in, something or someone you have complete faith in – what if that truth you live by turned out to be a lie? What if that person you trusted with your health and wellbeing turned out to be a liar? Let's imagine such a person for a moment. Let's create a fictitious person in our minds that is initially so convincing, so inspirational, that you can't help but be charmed by them. To begin with, they seem to want nothing from you, only support. They've been through tough times themselves. They're not setting themselves up as better than you, far from it. They're like you, they are you. They understand your frustrations, your issues, your hopes and fears and dreams. They've been where you've been. They've been ill and searched for a cure, or they've been unhealthy and searched for wellness. They are the projection of everything you want in one charming package. And they are here to help you. Or are they?'

After that, it's my turn. We're going to share this speech all the way through, a paragraph each.

'So,' I begin, 'let's create our perfect wellness scammer. Let's call her Julie.'

Oh, if I could see Clio's face right now. But I mustn't. I must look ahead at our audience. And I can see, they're rapt. There's a frisson in the air. Nobody knows quite what's going on but I can feel in the audience a tingling sense that we're up to something. And it's terrifying me. What Tara and I are doing is risky as hell. I have no idea what the outcome will be. But we're deep into it now and there's no turning back. My mouth goes horribly dry. I can't swallow properly; my tongue feels like wire wool. And at that moment, the door goes and in comes a couple of latecomers. And I can see it is Jacqui and her son Harvey! They must've finished the hospital appointment and made it after all! I'm so happy to see them! They creep in and find a couple of spaces on the second row. Seeing my bestie and her gorgeous lad give me the strength to go on.

'So, Julie is poorly. She's really poorly. She's so poorly, she's got the worst poorliness most of us could ever imagine. It's a disease that kills a lot of us, and a lot of our loved ones, our friends, neighbours and colleagues. Treatment is brutal, survival is not guaranteed. And Julie tells us, she knows. She's been through it. And she came out the other side and survived. She tells us that this disease is an enemy, a foe we must defeat. She talks in terms of battles that we must win or lose. And nobody wants to be a loser, do they? So, we must fight this enemy. And we must win. But the medical establishment can only offer treatments that make you feel worse than the disease itself. What's the sense in that?! Never mind that the treatment often works. But Julie convinces you it's poison they're putting in you! Julie has a better idea. She tells you that anything touted by hospitals and people in white coats is bad for you. It's scientific. It's modern. It's not natural. It's not old knowledge. It's not to be trusted.'

Tara goes on:

'So, Julie will share with you the secrets of the treatment plan she's come up with. Little Julie, out there, taking on scary Big Pharma and nasty western medicine, all on her own, a singular voice against the storm of convention. She took them all on . . . and she won! She made protein smoothies, she cooked organic wholefoods, she drank coconut water and ate seaweed and who knows what else. We don't know because you need to pay her to find out what else she did. She's not giving away her secrets for free. After all, she has to make a living. You can't begrudge her that. So everything Julie says and does is monetised. She's helping the world – a tenner at a time. You can be privy to the secrets of her success – for hundreds of pounds, even thousands. And never fear, she'll make sure some of it goes to charity, but you never see that money again, you don't know what it was spent on, you never hear from the charities it was supposed to go to, and you don't even know if the money was sent to those charities at all.'

I'm watching the audience. People are starting to look at Clio. It's happening. Just like Tara and I planned.

My turn again:

'Julie's bank balance is swelling now. Growing bigger and bigger by the day. She says wise things, she makes you feel special. You'll pay more to hear more from her. She knows things you don't know. She's more beautiful than you are, she's cooler, she has better hair and skin and clothes and shoes. She is everything you want to be. And she knows it. She knows how to flatter you. She asks you to fill in a detailed questionnaire about yourself, your family and your medical history, before you see her. She has all the details she needs. So when you're with her, she knows how to manipulate you, your thoughts, your feelings, the right questions to ask, to steer you, to guide you to think about the things she wants you to, she knows from all that private information you've willingly given her exactly what buttons to press, exactly which seeds to plant in your mind, that will lead to your vulnerabilities, the things that make you sad or glad, the things that she can bend to make you feel as if she's provided you with all the answers. She's clever. Oh, so clever, is our Julie. She listens, she processes, she moulds you like a pot on a wheel. And you come out of there feeling like you've had a revelation. And maybe you have. Maybe some of the things that Julie does and says actually help you. If it were all nonsense, she wouldn't get repeat visits, she wouldn't hook you in. She has to make you feel like the big chunks of money you're spending are worth it. So that you'll spend more. And more. And more. She's no fool.'

Tara's turn now:

'So, now you're hooked. You've got the app, you're donating to the charities, you go to the pricey retreats at swanky hotels, you go for therapy every week, you buy the products on Julie's website that she recommends and receives affiliate money from. You're doing everything she wants and you're feeling better than ever. For a while. But then . . . the rot sets in. The juices and the talking cure aren't actually making you any better. It's not changing your life. Your old habits are hard to break at first, and you did break them, with Julie's advice, and you went great guns for a while. But your illness doesn't actually get any better. Your aches don't go away. Your disease doesn't cure itself. Your psychic pain is still there. You can't keep it up, all this stuff you're pouring into your body and your brain. Because real life is always there to drag you back to reality. And you start to doubt this miracle cure now. Because it's not working. Because it never was going to work. Because it never did work for Julie in the first place. Because she made the whole thing up.'

An audible gasp from the audience. They're onto us now. They know what we're doing. They're looking at Clio now, I can see their eyes trained on her, then back to us.

I go on:

'That's right, Julie is a liar. She was never ill. She never had the disease, the one that you had, or your mum had, or your brother, or your boss or your best friend. She pretended to have it. She told you she had one disease and told another client she had another, whichever disease you had experience of, she'd had it too. She made you feel, wow, what a coincidence! Or maybe it was meant to be, that you have this connection. But people talk. Her clients start chatting. And they realise she told you all different things, whatever worked best for you and the experiences you've had, she told you what you wanted to hear. I had that, she said. I understand, she said. And when you start asking questions, when you start to challenge her, she panics. And she tells you, the disease has come back. She's golden now. Nobody can verbally attack someone with a disease. Imagine the bad karma! You'd get cancelled! Or sued! She's the victim now, ill again, after all this time. The tragic angel of wellness. But it's all bullshit. She starts a blog on her website, a journal of her fake disease, she takes fake selfies of herself in hospital, admitting herself to A&E under false pretences to get pics, or ordering a bunch of medical paraphernalia off Amazon and setting up a bed at home, with a white flannel sheet behind, and a fake port taped to her hand to look like a drip. But if you look really carefully, on the edge of the picture, you can see there's a strip of wall beside the white sheet she hung up to look like a hospital wall. It's not even a hospital. It's the stone walls of her house where you went to therapy. You'd know those walls anywhere. She's clever, is our scammer Julie, but she's not infallible, especially when she knows you're onto her and she's on the run. She makes clumsy mistakes, as we all do. Because it turns out, she's not special. She's not wiser than you. She's not more "well" than you. It's all fake. And lies. And a scam. She tricked you. And you fell for it. And now you feel like a loser all over again. And Julie won.'

And now, I can't help myself, as Tara continues, I take

the quickest glance at Clio's face. And oh, it's a picture. Her perfect skin doesn't look so perfect now. Her cheeks are burning with fury! And I bet her ears are burning too. Because only an idiot couldn't see the comparison, that we're talking about her. But we don't use her name, not even her real name, Julia. And we don't mention cancer. Or past-life regression. Or any identifying details. Tara made sure of that. Clio is squirming in her seat! And that is priceless.

Chapter 30

Tara takes up the baton and carries on, as I bask in the memory of Clio's delicious discomfort:

'But you're not alone. We all fall for this rubbish. Even trusted companies do. Even CEOs. And directors. And managers and assistants and cleaners and all of us. We're all susceptible. We all want to be well, don't we? But think about it: how well can a person be? It sets up a state of constant competition. Scroll through the wellness hashtag on Instagram and you'll see image after image after image of people engaging in wellness activities like it's the Wellness Olympics. How many miles can you run before work? How many anti-inflammatory fruits and veg can you fit into one smoothie? How big can your biceps be and how muscly can your fanny muscles actually get?'

This causes a ripple of gasps and guffaws. I wrote that line – hehehe . . .

Tara pauses perfectly for comic timing, then goes on:

'It's exhausting just looking at it. And it's pricey. Make

no mistake, wellness is almost exclusively for those who can afford it. But it's not only about looking good on the outside. There's something about the wellness schtick that washes you inside and out, and I'm not talking about colonic irrigation. I'm talking about moral virtue. The wellness industry lines up your physical health alongside your moral health. A healthy person is a good person. Wellness equals good. And in this way, illness isn't even the opposite of wellness: instead not trying hard enough becomes equated with non-wellness, i.e. you're lazy, unmotivated, less morally sound. A quitter. A failure. A loser. Unless . . . '

My turn and I'm hitting my stride now, making my points and barely looking at the script, as I know exactly what I want to say to my staff about wellness now:

'Unless you spend the money and buy the thing and then yay! You're a winner again, a better body, a better life, a better person. The worst thing about the wellness industry is that it can separate us from others, not bring us together. It pits us against each other, not providing a true community. It praises the individual, it warns you not to trust the medical establishment at all, to "do your own research" and by this they mean watch more TikToks or Instagram Reels, using "anecdotal evidence" as prime and outplaying any scientific evidence. It pretends to worship ancient ways but so often with a vast lack of actual knowledge of the cultural history it's trying to appropriate, creating the deeply flawed ideal that anything old is good and new is bad. Herbalism good, medication bad. And don't get me wrong, in western medicine, each medicine and surgery and treatment has its place and some work well and others don't work so well, for different people with different bodies. And the same goes for more ancient knowledge. Some will work and some won't, for different people. And you can do your own research into medical advice, and it could absolutely help you, as long as you find multiple, trusted sources, not some idiot on Insta. But the idea that all medicine is inherently bad and more so-called natural ways of living are inherently good is also deeply flawed. It means that a twenty-five-year-old in athleisurewear on Instagram knows more about your polycystic ovary syndrome than a fifty-five-year-old gynaecologist does, or some bloke who eats raw liver for breakfast every day knows more about your prostate than your GP does. And these untrained, unqualified scammers can flog you the magic beans to cure all your ills. It creates a falsely level playing field. We all know that doctors mess up and get things wrong, sometimes they don't listen or they assume and presume too much. But let's not pretend that a young adult making smoothies knows more than they do or even more than we ourselves know. These influencers are self-appointed experts, using numbers of followers as their kudos when underneath, we all know that's fake too.'

I glance over at Nick, who still looks entirely bemused by the whole thing. Then I look at Derek, whose face is completely different from how I imagined it would be. He looks pale. And he's not looking at me. He's looking down at the front row, at his wife, at Janey. I look at her and she's sitting there with her mouth open, drinking in every word. Oh, thank God. I really think we might've pulled it off. Tara ramps up the drama, her voice getting louder and fiercer:

'And the more you watch that kid on Insta making smoothies, the more your algorithm shows you stuff like that, which feeds your new obsession in making yourself perfect. All of us – whoever you are, wherever you come from, whatever your age or gender or ethnicity or any other measure – you are susceptible to wellness scams. If you're a woman, you are more likely to be targeted by wellness scammers, as they know the fact that women are more likely to be overlooked and unheard by a male-dominated medical establishment and thus these charming female influencers are approachable and they listen and they sympathise, not like the cold medical staff in their white coats. While if you're a man, you're more likely to be targeted by the manosphere, that place where you're led to believe that masculinity is under attack, that there is such a thing as an alpha male and whatever the hell that is, you're not that and thus you're a failure. Wellness scammers are healthy and wealthy and beautiful and wise. We want to *be them* and we want them to *be our* best friend. Googling wellness is a chaotic mess of misinformation and disinformation. Where do we even start? What can we trust? The influencer will assert – *me*. *You can trust me*, they tell us. Wellness influencers create problems you didn't even know you had and then provide the solution, usually at great expense that is funnelled directly from your hard-earned cash into their own pockets. And the winner is . . . the scammer. And definitely not you. Never you. The house always wins.'

It's my turn to bring this baby home now. I don't look at Clio, or Nick, or Derek. I look at my bestie, Jacqui, sitting there with her poorly son. She sees my gaze and punches a fist in the air. I punch one back. There's a reaction in the crowd. People are whispering excitedly. My staff are watching me intently. As I pause, you could hear a pin drop.

'So, my friends. My staff, who I've worked with day in, day out, for all these years. Today was about introducing our new wellness policy. And I want to tell you that I deeply care about how well you are, how good you feel about your job, and how we can help you feel better. Because we spend far more time at work than out of it. We see our work colleagues far more than we see our own families. That's crazy, when you think about it. But it's the system we have and we have to do our best with the system we're in. So, what does workplace wellness really mean? Whatever it is, I'm telling you now, that my belief is, whatever we're looking for, it will not be found in the wellness industrial complex. It won't be found in the Julies and all those like her, who tout their secrets for hard cash. That's the thing with the wellness industry: you can't win. You can't reach perfection. The wellness industry tells you that you need this, and you need that, and you should want this, and want that, forever and ever, amen. They'll keep flogging you this jar or box or bottle of stuff, or this treatment or procedure or therapy to attend, because you're never, ever going to be good enough to just BE YOURSELF. The wellness industry scams us all by making us live up to impossible standards, making us lie to ourselves about being better, healthier, thinner, harder working, harder playing, impossibly happy and just perfect, perfect, PERFECT.

'But the whole thing is a lie. Life isn't about being competitively more well than anyone else. Life is about people, all the people who make life worth living. And being okay with who you are, because in this cult of wellness, self-love becomes an obsession that crowds out all others and let's face it, while we're all obsessed with ourselves and how cleansed our internal organs are or how magnetised our auras are or whatever, we don't collectivise, we don't question, we don't debate, we don't celebrate life in all its complexity and all its contradictions, and all the people out there who challenge us and surprise us. We just turn inwards. There's nothing wrong with self-care. And not beating yourself up. Wellness isn't complicated. It isn't an obtuse secret that only the initiated know. You don't have to be Dr Strange to learn the secrets of the universe. It's common sense. You know this stuff already. Go for more walks, eat some good stuff that you know makes your tummy happy, get more sleep, see more friends, get more sunlight on your skin and try out activities that make you feel great, like a bit of yoga or rugby or swimming or sword-fighting or whatever the hell you want, whatever gets your body moving and you having fun. Get a massage if that makes you feel good, see a Reiki healer or a reflexologist if that truly helps you. It's your body, your mind and your choice. Care for your damn self. But self-care means nothing if you don't pay it forward. Don't listen to the scammers who want to make you feel fake special for a quick buck. Look after yourself and look after your fellow humans – your friends, your family, your neighbours, your work colleagues and the average human on the street or anywhere in the world you don't even know. Because being director of HR for all these years has taught me one essential truth about life: that *people* matter. That *you* matter.'

And we're done. And the moment the crowd realises that, it erupts. Jacqui and Harvey stand up, and so does Janey, and that encourages the rest and soon everyone is on their feet. They're clapping their hands like mad and stamping their feet and cheering and laughing and gossiping and having a great time. And in the midst of all that, Clio Kenton gets up and does the one thing that will make her look most guilty: she strides across the stage behind us and rushes down the steps and more or less sprints to the exit door. And she's outta here! And that little performance brings a whoop and more laughter from the crowd. Everyone knows now, everyone understands now. I can see it in their faces and I can hear it in their applause. We did it. I turn to Tara and give her a big hug and the crowd lap it up! Then Tara turns to the crowd and doesn't wait for them to quieten down. She just says, very loudly, right into her mic: 'Bar's open and the drinks are on Derek!'

That raises an even bigger cheer!

But now . . . it's time for Tara and for me to face the music.

We walk over to the CEOs, Clio's empty seat left forlornly between them. Derek might well have had a revelation about Janey's treatment during our speech. But for now, he's been humiliated. And he's mad. He's really mad.

'Have you any idea, the two of you, the damage that you've done today? Have you? Have you any comprehension of how much hot water this has placed us in? You probably thought you were being heroic and clever. Oh, the clever little women, saving the day!'

Jesus. Derek is really showing his true colours now. And to be honest, I'm listening to every word he spits at us and something strange is happening to me. I realise that I just . . . don't . . . care. I don't care what Derek says or does now. I feel like this enormous weight has lifted from me. Even when Derek jabs his finger in our direction and finishes with this:

335

'And you're both fired! Both of you! Fired! Do you hear me?!'

'Actually, you're not.'

Who's that? A voice behind Derek turns out to be Nick Bridges. He comes to stand beside Derek, who looks at him viciously.

'Sorry, Derek, but I became CEO at midday today, as agreed in my contract. And these two directors have done their job brilliantly. It's come to my attention that you were approached last night by your director of HR, who presented you with evidence that your hire for director of workplace wellbeing was most likely a confidence trickster. Instead of taking your director's concerns seriously and doing your own due diligence by looking into this new hire's credentials before hiring her for a senior post within our highest level of management – without my knowledge, I may add – you have laid us open to countless problems down the line. However, as it happens, we will be able to solve this issue. Our head of legal has told me everything and I agree with her – and our director of HR – that Clio Kenton's contract will not be going ahead. Our legal expert will see to that. Tara informed me of everything first thing this morning, taking all the blame on herself for introducing the wellness bootcamp and Clio to Lucy and to the company. And not only that, but Tara also informed me that a local journalist is the one whose expert research has tracked down Clio Kenton's suspicious past and present behaviour and thus I invited her here today to meet with me, and Tara, and Lucy to see what we can do together to rectify this situation. In fact, the journalist Jacqui Palmer has emailed me this afternoon to inform me that one of the charities that Clio Kenton claimed to be paying has been in touch with her this morning and is seeking to bring legal action against Clio Kenton for misappropriation of charity funds. Since it now appears that criminal proceedings may well be in motion against Clio Kenton, she has already broken clauses in her contract about bringing Beane & Co into disrepute and thus her contract is likely to already be null and void. In the meantime, the brilliant speech of our two directors here – and its direct result with Clio literally running from this room – has sorted our staff morale and halted all speculation about our new appointee. Everybody at Beane & Co is now in no doubt that their directors put their staff's needs first, even risking humiliation to do so. Our staff morale today has probably never been higher. All that's needed now is a meeting this afternoon between myself, our venerable directors of HR and legal, as well as our local journalist, where we shall consider the evidence gathered so far, thrash this out and make decisions as to the best course of action. Thus, Lucy and Tara, I have yet more news for you both. You're not fired. In fact, you're both promoted to the post of COO as of now. I've decided to award you both the same role, with a substantial pay rise for you both, as Beane & Co needs you both. Together you'll oversee the operation of the company and direct its future, as well as continuing to oversee the direction of your specialisms of the legal side of things, in Tara's case, and the brilliant management of our people, in Lucy's case. That is the only restructure I recommend at this time. So there will be no job losses for our staff and I just know that my two new COOs will face the future together as a great team. Lastly, I want to thank Derek for his decades of service and wish him all the very best in his retirement with his wonderful wife Janey. I'm sure you'd like to join with me in congratulating Derek on his achievements and wishing him a happy and healthy future.'

Wow. That was a speech and a half. We're all dumbstruck! Literally, three of the most loquacious people in the whole company have literally no words. Derek looks baffled but senses that he's off the hook and officially retired now, so whatever tricksy legal things might be ahead, he doesn't have to deal with it. Tara offers him her hand and congratulates him. I know I should do the same but my mind and body feel absolutely frozen. This is the moment I've been waiting for. The objective of all my efforts over years and years and years, day in, day out, at Beane & Co, battling with difficult staff, protecting decent staff, doing my CEO's bidding and flogging myself every week to fulfil and go beyond in every aspect of my work life. And now I have it, after all this time, the very thing I wished for.

'Congratulations to you too, Tara,' says Derek, still looking a little dazed. 'And to you, Lucia. Well deserved.'

'It's Lucy,' I say, my voice a whisper, having lost so much moisture after that mammoth speech that the inside of my mouth resembles the film set of *Dune*.

'Sorry?' says Derek. 'Come again?'

'My name is Lucy,' I say, far louder than I intended.

'It is indeed,' says Nick Bridges and holds out his hand. 'Congratulations on your promotion to the role of COO, Lucy. You've more than earned it.'

I stare at him, then glance at Derek, then Tara, then look behind me and, now that most of the staff have repaired to the bar, I can see Jacqui and Harvey waiting patiently and chatting. Jacqui sees me and waves, grinning. I lift my hand

and wave back. I feel hypnotised. Because something has occurred to me. It happened at the very moment Nick told me about my promotion. Something clicked in my head, like a cog slotting into place. A realisation. An epiphany.

'Thank you, Nick, for this fantastic opportunity,' I say.

'You're more than welcome,' he says with his customary confident smile.

'But I'm going to have to decline. I'm handing in my notice today. Thank you again for this opportunity. But also, I'm going to have to say . . . no, thank you.'

EPILOGUE

A few weeks on, I look back on that day of the conference and it feels like a vision from one of Clio's sessions. Sometimes I can't believe it happened, I can't believe Tara and I really did that. But it did happen. And yes, I did turn down that promotion. It wasn't planned. I had no idea I was going to say that to Nick Bridges. After all, I had everything I'd wanted: a new job at a higher level, better money, a new friend in Tara to work with who I genuinely trust and like . . . but you know what? I decided in that moment that if this wellness bullshit has taught me anything, it's that life is too short to carry on in old patterns, walking down worn-out ruts of behaviour and expectation. I want to walk in another direction. I turned down the job because I want to follow a new road: I want to make my own, new desire path. I know I'll have left my beloved company of Beane & Co in good hands with Tara and that we'll keep in touch as friends. The day of the staff conference was my last day. Nick agreed to an immediate notice, since my other staff in HR had been so well trained by me that they were able to step up and do my job, until a new director of HR had been appointed. It was the strangest thing, waking up the Monday morning after that weekend and knowing I had nowhere to go and nothing to do. I spent a couple of weeks just sleeping, and eating croissants along with a good range of rainbow foods and even a smoothie or two, and reading biographies of kings and queens in bed, and watching historical documentaries and black-and-white movies, and doing a bit of living-room yoga, and getting out in the spring sunshine and walking in lovely, ancient places, and visiting Dad's grave and dishing all the gossip. It's been heaven.

So, no more corporate bullshit for me. No more looking after staff wellbeing all the time – I've done that with bells on and done my time for those folk at the company. Tara will look after them. And I will always have my bestie Jacqui. The best news of all is two-fold: she's taken Harvey to see a private rheumatologist who is actually good and actually listened, which not all consultants do. And he's made a treatment plan for Harvey which looks like it will help that lovely boy. The other fab thing is that Jacqui is busy writing up her article about Clio and has applied for a new job at a bigger newspaper and has an interview next week, which I know she'll smash. In other news, Clio has gone to ground. Word on the grapevine is that she's stopped all her therapy sessions and more or less disappeared. Her website has gone from the internet. Once Jacqui's article is published, and the charities have finished their investigations, what we've heard is that it's very likely criminal proceedings will be brought against her. In even better news, Derek's wife Janey has a date set for surgery and after that will start undergoing chemo. It's not easy – cancer never is, for heaven's sake – but at least she's getting the treatment she needs. Janey actually sent me a letter, thanking me, Tara and Jacqui for our help. That brought a tear to my eye. And I bloody hope once news of Clio's doings gets out, once Jacqui publishes and – one fine day – a criminal trial hopefully begins, all of Clio's other clients who followed her dangerous advice will seek better treatment too. We can but hope.

So, life is moving on, for all of us. Good things are happening. My bestie is happy, my company is sorted. As for me, I don't know what I'm going to do next, in my working life. The only thing I know for sure is that I'll go to New Zealand first, spend some time with my mum, my sister and her husband, and my nephews. My family. After that, I really have no idea. Maybe I'll stay in New Zealand. Maybe I won't. Maybe I'll visit every ancient place in the world I've ever read about and never been to. Maybe I'll start up my own business somewhere. I've got those hard-earned savings, so I'm going to take a breather and I now have faith that my future will come to me when I'm ready. Now it's time for me to meet some new people and see what else is out there. That, to me, is the definition of wellness: being true to yourself, yet also opening your life up to possibility. And off I go! It's time to live, laugh and fuck off.

ACKNOWLEDGEMENTS

Huge thanks for help during the writing of this book goes to: Janey Stevens, for giving her time for an extensive interview about Reiki & wellness.

Early readers, Lucy Adams & Pauline Lancaster, for always giving such helpful and generous feedback.

Everyone who responded to a Facebook post about wellness from 4 November 2024: Trish Colton, Tracey Edges, Effie Merryl, Michael Packman, Eleanor Small and Eileen F. Wharton.

Emma Graham Tallon, for her very helpful message about acupuncture.

Rachel Hart, for choosing wellness, for detailed help on early research and for always being spot on about the zeitgeist.

Laura Macdougall and Eleanor Horn at United Agents, my brilliant agent team, for steering this author's career over the many bumps in the road.

Katie Sadler and Sam Missingham, for excellent advice on

marketing and Lucy McCarraher, for inviting me to speak and for supporting my writing career so kindly.

Anna Nightingale and all of the team at Avon, for their fabulous vision for all Harper Ford books.

Readers, book bloggers and reviewers on Facebook, Instagram, TikTok and wherever you reside, for such wonderfully enthusiastic support for Harper Ford books and awesome posts and pics.

Friends and family, including my Facebook fam, for their unending support especially when my own precarious wellness decides to get lost.

Ginette Fairall, for her generosity and kindness.

My Auntie Biddy – Bridget Ash – for her wonderful support for all things Harper Ford.

Kitty Wilson and Sarah Waights, for the long chats and listening to me rattle on and rant.

Fiona McKinnell and Sue White, for looking after me in every way a friend might need.

Emma Pass and Maureen Burdock, for being brilliant writer buddies.

As ever, Poppy, Clem and Tink, for living, laughing and never leaving me lonely.

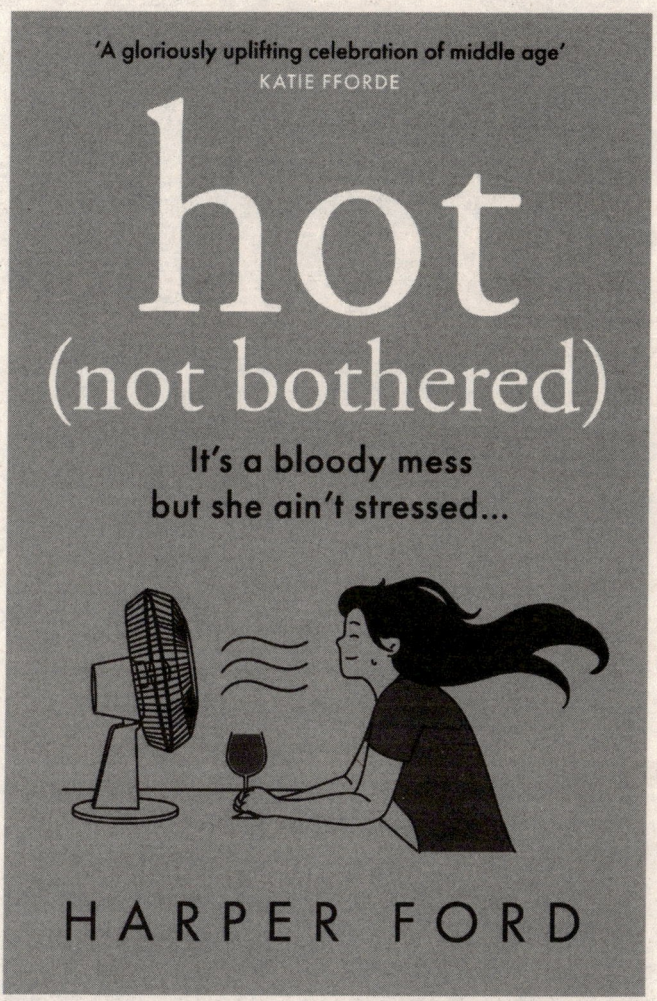

hot
(not bothered)

It's a bloody mess
but she ain't stressed...

HARPER FORD

Don't miss the hilarious, uplifting and relatable
menopause romcom, perfect for fans of Alexandra
Potter, Sophie Kinsella and Fiona Gibson!

It's a bloody mess but she ain't stressed. . .

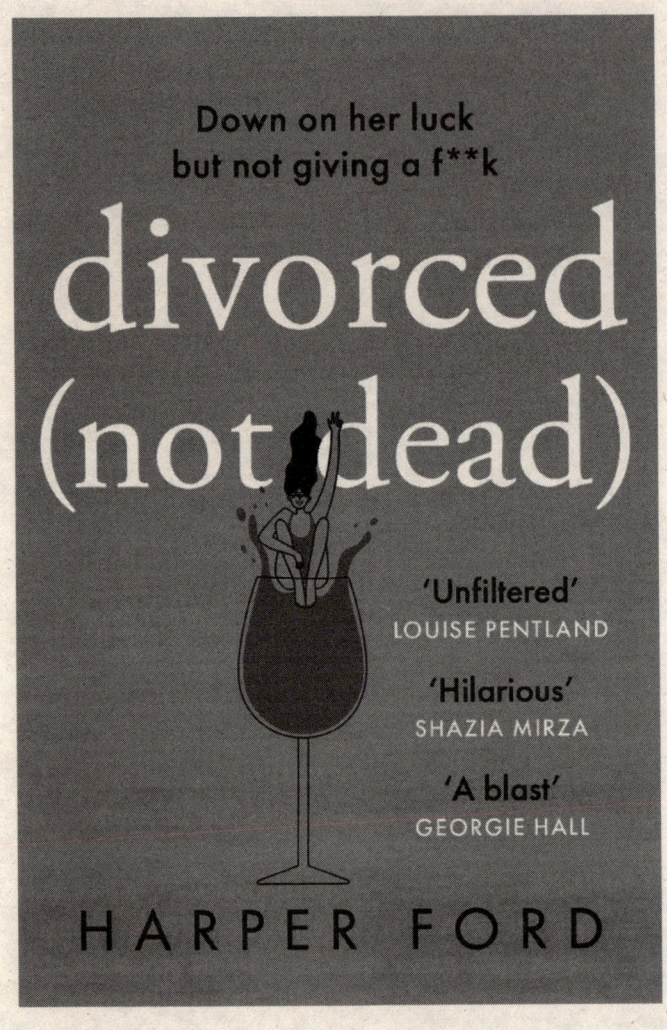

Down on her luck
but not giving a f**k

divorced
(not dead)

'Unfiltered'
LOUISE PENTLAND

'Hilarious'
SHAZIA MIRZA

'A blast'
GEORGIE HALL

HARPER FORD

Fans of Alexandra Potter, Marian Keyes and Caroline
James will love *Divorced Not Dead*,
a no-holds-barred, heartfelt and laugh-out-loud
hilarious romcom about being fifty,
but absolutely not yet dead yet!